the ADRENAL STRESS connection

The Adrenal STRESS Connection
Second edition

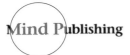

Our focus is education

FOR INFORMATION CONTACT

Mind Publishing Inc.
PO Box 57559
1031 Brunette Avenue
Coquitlam, BC Canada V3K 1E0
Tel: 604-777-4330 Toll free: 1-877-477-4904
Fax: 1-866-367-5508
Email: info@mindpublishing.com
www.mindpublishing.com

ISBN: 978-1-927017-20-3
Printed in Canada.

Disclaimer:
This publication contains the ideas and opinions of its authors. It is intended to provide helpful and informative material on the subjects addressed in the publication. It is sold with the understanding that the authors and the publisher are not engaged in rendering medical, health, or any other kind of personal professional services in the book. The reader should consult his or her medical, health, or other competent professional before adopting any of the suggestions in this book or drawing inferences from it.

The authors and publisher specifically disclaim all responsibility for any liability, loss, or risk, personal or otherwise, which is incurred as a consequence, directly or indirectly, of the use and application of any of the contents of this book.

Contents

Foreword

Adrenal fatigue is a very common and quickly growing problem of modern life. The stressors we are faced with on a daily basis, such as family and financial problems, increased work load, lack of physical exercise, insufficient rest, poor diet and environmental toxins all contribute to more stress on the stress adaptive organs, the adrenal glands. Adrenal stress has left millions of people suffering from a problem that mostly goes unrecognized and untreated. Not only does the undiagnosed condition cause financial losses for individuals and companies through worker absenteeism but also the individual experiencing the problem can no longer experience life to his or her full capacity due to the various symptoms of adrenal fatigue. In addition, people suffering from adrenal fatigue are much more likely to develop various other common diseases ranging from diabetes, cancer, heart disease and more which we will cover in this book.

I (Dr. Jensen) was first introduced to my adrenal glands over thirty years ago. I was a single mom with three children under three years of age, newborn twin sons and a three-year-old son. My marriage had recently dissolved and I was working full time as a teacher for learning and behavioral problem adolescents. Well as you can imagine, it didn't take long for me to hit the wall with such an extreme fatigue that I didn't know what to do. The medical doctors could find nothing wrong and out of desperation I went to see the local naturopath. He told me that I had adrenal fatigue and put me on a health program to support these stress organs that were no longer doing a good job at adapting to the stressors in my life. I was back to my normal energy quite quickly but I also realized that I would probably need to be on and off adrenal support throughout my life as the level of stress wasn't about to change any time soon. At the time I had no idea that in the future I would end up studying to be a naturopathic physician and that learning more about the importance of adrenal health would become one of my life's passions. Now for over 25 years in clinical practice, I have seen in my patients the incredible results of supporting the adrenal glands. Our purpose of this book is to give you, the reader, enough information so that you can take the necessary steps to help you recover from the symptoms or conditions caused by adrenal fatigue.

The first time I (Dr. Schauch) learned about adrenal stress was in naturopathic school: my colleagues and I had no idea that we were on our way to adrenal burn out. When I started my practice, I was amazed at how these two small glands had the ability to control sleep, appetite, inflammation, digestion, anxiety/depression, hormones and much more. I soon realized that these glands were so vitally important to our health. It is now standard in my practice, even if patients reassure me that "they have no stress," to test the adrenal glands. I have seen year after year, patients improve when adrenal health is restored. Studies have revealed that stress experienced even in your mother's womb can affect the function of your adrenal glands later on in life. We hope that you find this book helpful in identifying your adrenal stress connection in order to create a superior and healthier you.

Acknowledgments

Dr. Jensen's Acknowledgments

We would like to thank Deane Parkes for his commitment to educating the public about how to obtain and maintain optimal health. One of the things on my "bucket list" was to publish a book on adrenal health – and here we are – Thank you, Deane!

Thank you to Dr. Marita Schauch, ND, for her energy, for being so enthusiastic about contributing to this book and for her passion for educating her patients and the public about the importance of adrenal health. It is so nice to see this passion carried forward.

My three sons are the greatest gift in my life and I am forever grateful for all of the lessons and the love in our journey together.

My patients over the years have been the fuel for the fire that has kept my passion alive in the field of medicine. It was an honor to be part of their healing journey and it was the empathetic listening to my patients that kept me in touch with the reality of medical practice; the patient experience versus the mountains of statistics.

Writing this book is yet another reminder that nothing can be accomplished in my life without the support and knowledge of others and the guidance and grace of something bigger than myself – *Divine Spirit*.

Dr. Schauch's Acknowledgments

Thank you to my loving family; my husband Markus, mom and dad and brother Mike for all your love, support, guidance and encouragement.

Thank you to Dr. Karen Jensen for allowing me to transform my passion for adrenal health into this amazing book, a vision that I have always had.

To my friend, Doug Muldoon, through his connections, else this would never have come to be.

To my patients who have challenged and taught me to be a better doctor every day in practice.

CHAPTER 1

The Adrenal Stress Connection

"States of health or disease are, at the heart, the organism's success or failure at adapting to environmental challenges." – RENÉ DUBOS

One of the characteristic features of all living beings is their ability to maintain the constancy of their internal milieu despite changes in their surroundings. Whenever this self-regulating power fails, disease or even death occurs. Truly, life is largely a process of adaptation to the circumstances in which we live, and the secret of health and happiness lies in our successful adjustment to the ever-changing conditions created by the world around us and by our inner search for truth. The greater our self-knowledge on all levels, and the greater our willingness to take responsibility for our own lives and expressing our truth, the greater will be our ability to adapt to and embrace life.

The great majority of illnesses have a number of causes and one of the main causes of ill health is the effect of stressors on those self-regulating balances.

Surveys and research reports indicate that approximately 45% of all adults suffer adverse effects to stress while 75-90% of all visits to physicians are in some way related to the results of psychosocial stress. Stress is a factor in many illnesses – from headaches to heart disease, immune deficiencies, anxiety disorders and digestive problems, just to name a few.

In today's fast-paced society, the vast majority of individuals are under a barrage of constant stressors. While some of the initial fight-or-flight stress responses may be beneficial to survival (acute stress), there is an increased risk of various physical and psychological health challenges when the stressors are prolonged (chronic stress). Stress is not going away and it is not something new. However, in today's world of technological advances, we are seldom "unplugged" from the cell phone or laptop. Divorce rates hover near their highest in history, the concept of job security is gone by way of the dinosaur and time to just kick back, unplug and "smell the roses" is a concept that is fading. Stress has become endemic and it penetrates to the core of our being and changes us in the process, altering our bodies and our brains.

Some stress is absolutely normal and necessary in living creatures and everyone has a built-in gauge that helps control our reaction to various stressors. New research is indicating that the body can become "sensitized" to stress and the brain will re-circuit itself in response to stress. When this sensitization happens, the body just does not respond to stress the same way and the brain responds to a normal stress such as being late for an appointment as though it was a life-threatening event. Studies show that stressful events that occur in childhood, such as losing a parent or being raised by an alcoholic or abusive parent, can permanently rewire the brain's circuitry and result in inappropriate responses to stress.

The stress response is "wired" into our brain and even though we are no longer like the cave man running for our lives from the wild boar, studies have found that – for many – the same fight-or-flight stress circuits are all working overtime from varied stressors such as work deadlines, extreme weather, over-exercise, divorce or death of a loved one. Each of us is wired for stress differently and will have different responses to different stressors depending on our own unique wiring system.

Each of us will benefit from reducing stressors, but the obvious benefits will vary depending on our overall stress resistance capabilities, which are determined by our individual strengths and weaknesses.

Often, the stressors can be non-specific and less obvious and we may not be aware of the effects on our bodies and minds.

All living creatures are subject to stressors of internal and external origin and have the ability to respond to stressors.

WHAT ARE STRESSORS?

Stressors are events or situations – internal or external, pleasant or unpleasant – that require our body systems to adapt and respond in order to maintain balance, or homeostasis. When the stressor (regardless of its origin) is unrelenting, the body may lose its ability to adapt to it – the defense mechanisms become exhausted. Exhausted defense mechanisms are incapable of protecting the body and we become more susceptible to disease.

External Stressors

External stressors originate in our environment and include chemicals and other air, food and water pollutants, including radiation, as well as noise, weather changes and electromagnetic fields. We can diminish these external stressors once we have a better understanding of their sources and of how they are transmitted to us.

- **Weather and seasonal stressors.** These include overheating and overcooling, seasonal changes in weather and natural light patterns, and barometric shifts.
- **Chemical stressors.** The various forms of chemical stressors include toxic metals, persistent organic pollutants, junk food diets, alcohol, caffeine, tobacco, and both legal and illicit drugs.
- **Nutritional stress.** Modern agricultural and food processing practices have seriously depleted the nutritional content of most foods and pollutants contaminate the water supply.
- **Electromagnetic fields.** Sources include computers, cell phones, fluorescent lights, hair dryers, microwave ovens, power lines, televisions, waterbeds and anything else that is plugged in.

Weather and Seasonal Stress Reduction Tips:

- Go outside, without glasses on, for a minimum of one hour each day. You will get out of the toxic indoor office environment and increase your exposure to natural light.
- Use full-spectrum lighting wherever possible.
- If weather sensitive, support your adrenal glands with **AdrenaSense®**.

Nutritional Stress Reduction Tips:

- Consume whole foods such as organically grown, fiber-rich whole grains; fresh fruits and vegetables; and hormone- and chemical-free animal products.
- Limit consumption of refined carbohydrates (i.e., sugar, white breads, pasta)
- Avoid saturated fats, heated oils and margarines, fried foods and processed cooking oils. Increase your consumption of essential fatty acids.
- Increase your protein intake from vegetarian sources such as legumes and soy products.
- Increase your intake of green leafy vegetables.
- Drink only unfluoridated, unchlorinated water, and drink a minimum of 8-10 (8 ounce) glasses daily!
- Minimize or eliminate the consumption of soft drinks; drink beer and wine in moderation and spirits sparingly, if at all. Coffee and tea can be

taken in moderation, one to two cups daily at the most – they are diuretics and flush much-needed fluids from your body.

▶ AND take a good multivitamin/mineral supplement to buffer the deficiencies in our foods due to the above-mentioned reasons. Good quality vitamins that I would recommend are **Whole Earth & Sea™ Pure Food** supplements for women and men for additional nutritional insurance. Suggested use: 2 tablets per day.

MORE ON ENVIRONMENTAL TOXINS

Our environment is becoming increasingly more toxic each year from the air we breathe, harmful electromagnetic frequencies (EMFs), the food we eat and the water we drink. All of us are living with some degree of environmental toxins in our bodies. For many of us, these toxins are causing us to be ill and contributing to chronic disease.

These chemicals also create a very large toxic body burden and additional stress on our adrenal glands, immune system, hormonal pathways and detoxification organs such as the liver, kidneys and lymphatic system.

Facts:

▶ Each and every second 683 pounds of toxic chemicals are released into our air, land and water by industrial facilities around the world.

▶ This amounts to approximately 10 million tons (over 21 billion pounds) of toxic chemicals released into our environment by industries each year.

▶ Of these, over 2 million tons (over 4.5 billion pounds) per year are recognized carcinogens.

Chronic Disease is on the Rise

▶ Leukemia, brain cancer and other childhood cancers have increased by more than 20% since 1975.

▶ Asthma prevalence approximately doubled between 1980 and 1995 and has stayed at the elevated rate.

▶ Difficulty in conceiving and maintaining a pregnancy affected 40% more women in 2002 than in 1982. The incidence of reported difficulty has almost doubled in younger women ages 18–25.

▶ Since the early 1990s, reported cases of autism spectrum disorder have increased tenfold.

The last 30 years of environmental health science shows that small amounts of chemicals can have long-term effects when the exposure comes at vulnerable times of development. Studies have linked early life exposure to chemicals and the later diagnosis of breast cancer, learning and developmental disabilities, and Alzheimer's disease. A study published in Environmental Research (2013) measured prenatal exposure to BPA and found that this exposure was associated with internalizing behaviors, such as anxiety and depression in children.

The Environmental Working Group (EWG), an American environmental organization that specializes in research, tested umbilical cord blood samples from 10 babies born in U.S. hospitals. Tests revealed a total of 287 chemicals in the group! We will discuss the top 5 toxins below, many of which were found in the umbilical cord samples.

Xenoestrogens – What Are They?
Many of the chemicals we will be discussing below are classified as synthetic xenoestrogens. The word xenoestrogen is derived from the Greek words meaning "foreign estrogen." Xenoestrogens are clinically significant because they can mimic the effects of natural, endogenous estrogen produced in the body. They do this by blocking or binding to hormone receptors, which can be particularly detrimental to hormone sensitive organs such as the uterus and the breast, as well as our immune and neurological systems. Xenoestrogens can also alter estrogen and progesterone balance because as they enter the body they can increase the total amount of estrogen resulting in a condition known as "estrogen dominance." Xenoestrogens are particularly resilient and store in our fatty cells. The build-up of xenoestrogens has been implicated in many conditions including breast and prostate cancer, obesity, uterine fibroids, endometriosis, miscarriages, early onset puberty and menopause, and diabetes.

TOP 5 ENVIRONMENTAL TOXINS AND THEIR IMPACT ON OUR HEALTH
The first step to reducing the load of toxic buildup in our body is awareness and avoidance. Some of the main xenoestrogens in our environment are the following:

Bisphenol A (BPA)
BPA is a very common chemical found in plastics, food and beverage can linings, thermal receipts and other consumer products. BPA is known to mimic estrogen and studies have linked developmental exposure to BPA to reproductive harm, increased cancer susceptibility, and abnormalities in brain development and fat metabolism.

Tips to Avoid BPA Exposure

Although completely eliminating exposure to BPA may not be possible, there are steps you can take to reduce your family's exposure to this chemical by avoiding common sources and limiting exposure for the highest risk groups.

▸ The developing fetus and baby are the most vulnerable to BPA. Replace plastic sippy cups with glass or stainless steel.

▸ Do not microwave or store food or drink in plastic.

▸ Almost all canned foods sold in the United States and Canada have a BPA epoxy liner that leaches BPA into the food. The highest concentrations are found in canned meats, pasta and soups. Eden Foods uses an alternative technology for their canned beans but not for tomato-based products. Rinsing canned fruit or vegetables may reduce the amount of BPA you ingest.

▸ When possible, avoid polycarbonate, especially in children's food and drinks. This plastic may be marked with the recycling code #7 or the letters "PC." Plastics with the recycling labels #1, #2 and #4 on the bottom are better choices because they do not contain BPA.

▸ Avoid plastic reusable water bottles as well as metal food and beverage cans, including beer and soda cans as epoxy resins (BPA) are often used to coat the lining of these consumer products.

Dioxin

Dioxins are formed during waste burning, pulp and paper bleaching, and pesticide manufacturing. They can disrupt the delicate balance of both male and female sex hormone signaling in the body. Recent research has shown that exposure to low levels of dioxin in the womb and early in life can both permanently affect sperm quality and lower the sperm count in men during their prime reproductive years. Dioxins are also very long-lived and thus can build up both in the body and in the food chain.

Tips to Avoid Dioxin

More than 90% of human exposure is through food, mainly meat and dairy products, fish and shellfish.

▸ Dioxins and other chemicals store in fatty tissue so try to eat less animal fat – buy lean meats and poultry.

▸ Purchase food products that have been grass fed.

▸ Reduce your dairy consumption.

Atrazine

Atrazine is a herbicide used to prevent weeds in crops such as corn and sugar cane and on turf, such as golf courses and residential lawns.

It is one of the most widely used herbicides in the U.S. and was banned in the European Union in 2004 because of persistent groundwater contamination. As of 2001, Atrazine was the most commonly detected pesticide contaminating drinking water in the United States. Studies suggest that Atrazine is an endocrine disruptor and has been linked to breast tumors, delayed puberty and prostate inflammation in animals.

Tips to Avoid Atrazine
▸ Try to buy organic produce – check out the dirty dozen and the clean fifteen from www.ewg.org.
▸ Avoid tracking pesticides into the house by having everyone remove their shoes at the door.
▸ Vacuum carpets, mop floors, and damp-wipe dusty surfaces weekly, especially if you have small children who spend time on the floor.
▸ Filter your drinking water!

Phthalates

Phthalates are commonly found in plastics to make them more flexible and as lubricants in cosmetics. You will find phthalates in perfume, hair spray, deodorant and anything fragranced from shampoo to air fresheners to laundry detergent. They are also found in nail polish, carpeting, vinyl flooring, shower curtains and plastic toys.

Phthalates are known hormone disruptors and mimickers contributing to abnormal sexual development, obesity, and diabetes and thyroid irregularities.

Tips to Avoid Phthalates
▸ Avoid plastic food containers and plastic wrap made from PVC (recycling label #3).
▸ Some types of phthalates have now been banned from products such as children's toys and bottles, but these laws only took place in 2009, so avoid hand-me-down plastic toys.
▸ Stay away from fragrances. Instead use products that are scented with only essential oils without synthetic fragrance.
▸ Find phthalate-free personal care products with EWG's Skin Deep Data base: www.ewg.org/skindeep/

Perchlorate

Perchlorate is both a naturally occurring and man-made chemical used in the production of rocket fuel, missiles, fireworks, flares and explosives.

Perchlorate contaminates a good portion of our produce, water and milk. It is a major health concern because it can disrupt the thyroid's ability to produce hormones needed for normal growth and development. The U.S. Environmental Protection Agency (EPA) also states that perchlorate is considered a "likely human carcinogen."

Tips to Avoid Perchlorate
▸ Filter your water!
▸ Improve thyroid function by ensuring enough iodine in your diet.
▸ Try to buy organic as much as possible.

WHAT ABOUT HEAVY METALS?
Toxic metals such as aluminum, arsenic, mercury, cadmium and lead are often referred to as "heavy metals." These heavy metals from our environment are capable of accumulating in the body, especially in the brain, liver, kidneys, bone and immune system. Most of the heavy metals in the body are from contamination from industry. In the Unites States alone, industries dump more than 600,000 tons of lead into the atmosphere, which we either inhale or ingest from our food or water.

Sources of heavy metal toxicity include:
▸ Aluminum – aluminum-containing antacids, aluminum cookware, drinking water, some commercial vitamins (Centrum).
▸ Arsenic – drinking water, rice products
▸ Cadmium – cigarette smoke, drinking water
▸ Lead – car exhaust, dolomite, cosmetics, solder on tin cans, drinking water
▸ Mercury – dental amalgams (mercury fillings), drinking water, fish and shellfish

Signs and symptoms of heavy metal toxicity are usually vague. Mild cases may be associated with fatigue, headache and "brain fog" or loss of concentration and clarity. More severe cases may involve chronic pain, tremors, anemia, dizziness, poor coordination and other neurological symptoms.

WHAT IS EMF?
EMF stands for electromagnetic fields, which are a type of radiation that take place in the form of waves. There are two types of electromagnetic energy – natural EMFs and artificial EMFs. The earth produces an

electromagnetic field, and so does the human body. Natural EMFs are very low in intensity and research shows that every cell in the human body may have its own EMF to help regulate important functions and keep us healthy. Artificial EMFs such as cell phones, cordless phones, microwave ovens, baby monitors, GPS navigators and security systems create powerful high frequency EMFs that disrupt the body's natural energetic field. We are exposed to 100 million times greater artificial EMF radiation than our grandparents were, and that exposure grows each year.

Think about the stress that all these artificial EMFs put on the body as well as our stress glands – the adrenal glands. It is just another challenge that the body must deal with and adapt to. After an extensive review of 2000+ studies, the National Institute of Environmental Health Sciences concluded that EMFs "should be regarded as possible carcinogens" and potentially very harmful and toxic to our health. In today's world it is virtually impossible to avoid all artificial EMFs, but we can definitely work on minimizing our exposure.

Tips to Avoid EMFs

▶ Minimize your talk time on cell phones and try to eliminate calls over 20 minutes.
▶ Don't wear your cell phone like a pager – if your phone is turned on and worn on your belt or in a pocket you could be receiving a constant blast of radiation from the battery pack. Carry your cell phone in your purse or briefcase to minimize exposure.
▶ Minimize your time in front of the TV and computer.
▶ Don't use a microwave!

The book *A Wellness Guide for The Digital Age* by Kerry Crofton, PhD, is an excellent source of additional information as well as safer tech solutions for all things wired and wireless.

TOXIC STRESS

Many of the chemicals and toxins discussed in this chapter have been shown to impact physical and mental health. Long-term accumulation of chemicals has detrimental effects not only on our hormones but our adrenal stress response and organs of detoxification. How strong and healthy our bodies are will determine our ability to detoxify and eliminate these toxins.

Reducing Toxins Through Diet and Lifestyle

To reduce the load of environmental toxins, the first step is to stop carrying toxins into our homes and into our bodies. About 90% of our daily toxin intake comes from the air inside our homes and workplaces and the food that we eat. Some of us cannot make huge changes with the air quality at work, but we can definitely change the air in our homes.

Using high quality air filters that are changed regularly (every 6-8 weeks) is one of the best ways to reduce the toxin presence in your air at home. Opening the windows once a week when you are cleaning can bring in the fresh air and eliminate any accumulation of toxins. For those who are living in colder climates, bundle up and open the windows every few weeks and air out those pollutants and dust particles. Chemicals from outside (pesticides, heavy metals, etc.) are brought in from the soles of your shoes so remove your shoes before entering your house.

Another big source of toxin exposure as mentioned above is from the food we eat.

The Dirty Dozen and Clean Fifteen chart from www.ewg.org is an excellent guide for when you are grocery shopping. It outlines the fruits and vegetables with the highest pesticide residue versus those with the lowest pesticide residue.

The 12 MOST TOXIC fruits and vegetables include:
▶ Apples
▶ Strawberries
▶ Grapes
▶ Celery
▶ Peaches
▶ Spinach
▶ Sweet bell peppers
▶ Nectarines - imported
▶ Cucumbers
▶ Cherry tomatoes
▶ Snap peas – imported
▶ Potatoes

The CLEAN 15 fruits and vegetables include:
▶ Avocados
▶ Sweet corn
▶ Pineapples

- Cabbage
- Sweet peas – frozen
- Onions
- Asparagus
- Mangoes
- Papayas
- Kiwi
- Eggplant
- Grapefruit
- Cantaloupe
- Cauliflower
- Sweet potatoes

Pesticide and antibiotic residues in conventionally raised beef, dairy products and farmed fish (Atlantic salmon) should try to be eliminated. Organic and grass fed beef and dairy products should be encouraged. Certain fish also contain higher levels of mercury content such as shark, swordfish, king mackerel, tuna, marlin, halibut, snapper and lobster, and should be limited to once every 6-8 weeks.

Fish with the lowest mercury content include salmon, tilapia, sole, arctic char and clams. These types of seafood can be eaten 2-3 times per week.

Some Key Supplements

- ***Garlic*** improves circulation and has been shown to reduce blood pressure. Use liberally in foods or take as supplement.
  Suggested use: 1,000-3,000 mg/day

- ***Milk thistle*** (*Silybum marianum*) – The most impressive research showing support of liver function has been done on the extract of milk thistle. Milk thistle contains a group of flavonoids that promote liver health and also support the body's natural detoxification processes. This powerful herb supports the liver by acting as an antioxidant as well as prevents the depletion of glutathione. The antioxidant glutathione supports the liver and aids in the detoxification of harmful chemicals and toxins.
  Suggested use: 400-600 mg/day

▶ *Turmeric* (*Curcuma longa*) is a well-researched herb shown to have potent antioxidant and liver supportive properties. It also promotes healthy inflammatory responses.
Suggested use: up to 1500 mg/day

▶ *EstroSense*® gently supports the body's natural detoxification processes to help with healthy estrogen metabolism, the elimination of harmful toxins and prevention of toxic buildup in the body.
Suggested use: 2 capsules/day with food
***Milk thistle and turmeric as well as powerful detoxification nutrients and antioxidants such as I3C, DIM, calcium-D-glucarate, sulforaphane, green tea extract, lycopene and rosemary extract are all found in EstroSense.

▶ *AdrenaSense*® helps support and nourish healthy adrenal glands and thus reduce stress, especially when dealing with the environmental insult we are exposed to on a daily basis.
Suggested use: 2 capsules midday with food

▶ *Vitamin C* is a potent antioxidant and may also decrease lead levels. Vitamin C is also required for the synthesis of glutathione, which helps support our antioxidant defenses and prevent free radical damage from environmental toxins.
Suggested use: 1000-2000 mg/day with food

▶ *Probiotics* ensure healthy digestion and prevent the accumulation of harmful and "bad" bacteria. Having adequate "good" bacteria also helps the digestive system remove any harmful toxins through the bowels.
Suggested use: at least 10-20 billion CFUs/day with meals

INTERNAL STRESSORS

In our interactions with the environment, the inner and outer worlds continuously and reciprocally influence one another. Internal stress is frequently a direct result of modern life. Environmental toxins, improper diet, inappropriate use of drugs and hectic, sleep-deprived lifestyles all affect our nutritional status, intestinal health, and mental, emotional and spiritual health.

Life event stressors come in the form of cataclysmic events such as death of a loved one, an automobile accident or a serious illness. But stress can take its toll in less obvious ways like a bout of the flu, surgery, infected root canal, quarrels with loved ones, pressure in the workplace or living in an unhappy relationship, as well as other stress influences previously mentioned. Ongoing smaller stressors can be as equally harmful to the body as the more dramatic events.

Mental, Emotional and Spiritual Stress

"Visualization takes advantage of what might almost be called a "weakness" of the body: it cannot distinguish between a vivid mental experience and an actual physical experience." – BERNIE S. SIEGEL, MD

Once we fully understand that we do have choices in our lives, we come to realize that the majority of limitations we have are those we create with our own beliefs.

What we constantly imagine will become our individual reality. The more feeling there is behind the images, the more potently they are likely to manifest in the physical world. These concepts have a critical role to play in our journey to health. If our thought forms help to create our reality, we can use them to contribute to the creation of health – or of disease.

A continual focus on limiting beliefs, worries or unpleasant situations harms the physical body. I can't tell you how many times I hear people say such things as, "I get allergies every year at this time," "I worry myself sick about my children," or "I dread getting up in the morning because I hate my job." Thoughts like these do not just float around in the ethers; they create powerful effects on you and those around you. If you have enough destructive thoughts, they will result in physical, mental or emotional problems. Every thought, if strong enough, solidifies into a future condition.

Thoughts significantly affect everything in our lives, including our physiology and therefore our health. Our mental, behavioral and emotional responses have a profound effect on the fight-or-flight stress reaction.

Listen carefully to your spoken and unspoken thoughts and observe where they are leading you.

"In mechanical terms, the motor is the mind, but the fuel is the heart. Thus every thought combined with feeling brings into action certain physical tissue, parts of the brain, nerves or muscles. This produces an actual change in the conditions of the tissue, regardless of whatever body it be." – PAUL TWITCHELL

Mental, Emotional and Spiritual Stress Reduction Tips:
▶ Love is the essential healing force in the universe and brings us everything we need. Focus on how to express love or goodwill in every act and word, and love will return to you in abundance.
▶ Cultivate an attitude of gratitude for everything in your life. Look for the opportunity to learn and grow in every situation.
▶ Remember that thoughts – especially when accompanied by strong emotion – eventually manifest in physical reality. If you want to change your physical reality, change the focus of your thoughts. Especially replace disruptive, unpleasant, worrying and limiting thoughts with loving, liberating and forgiving thoughts.

The Serenity Prayer is a very gentle but powerful way to help someone maintain a state of mental peace. "God, grant me the serenity to accept the things I cannot change; the courage to change the things I can; and the wisdom to know the difference."

STRESS ADAPTATION

"To understand the mechanism of stress gives physicians a new approach to treatment of illness, but it can also give us all a new way of life, a new philosophy to guide our actions in conformity with natural laws." – HANS SELYE, MD

All individuals subjected to chronic and severe stress go through stages of adapting to these stressors. The stages of stress-induced damage were first studied by a Canadian doctor, Hans Selye. He gave us a greater understanding of how stress affects the entire body and, if stress is prolonged and severe, many people may develop adrenal insufficiency.

Dr. Selye calls the body's mechanism for dealing with stress the general adaptation syndrome (GAS). The GAS has three stages: (1) the alarm reaction, (2) resistance and (3) exhaustion.

Stage 1: *Alarm Reaction.* There is an initial reaction by the body to a stressor through a complex chain of physical and biochemical responses brought about by the interaction of the brain, nervous system and a variety of different hormones released through the main stress organs, the adrenal glands. In the initial fight-or-flight reaction to stress, the body goes on full alert and the adrenals produce extra stress hormones (hyperadrenic response). After the initial alarm reaction is over, the body goes into a recovery stage lasting 24-48 hours and the stress hormone levels return to normal. For instance, someone who works long hours on a project may come down with a cold or flu, and recover in a few days because the balancing mechanisms (stress adaptation abilities) are strong.

Stage 2: *Resistance.* In the resistance stage, the adrenal glands are on constant alert and over-secrete and over-react to prolonged stress. The main adrenal hormone at this point is cortisol, the hallmark of long-term stress. The resistance stage can last anywhere from a number of months to as much as 20 years. If the stress is unrelenting, eventually the adrenal glands will no longer be able to rebuild and adapt. The person gets a cold or flu, but instead of recovering after a few days of rest, they find the illness lingering for a much longer time. The body's ability to cope with stress has been lowered.

Stage 3: *Exhaustion.* In this phase, that state of hypoadrenia is to the point where the ability to respond to stress is severely limited. There are no reserves left for adapting to stressors, resulting in fatigue, malaise and lack of will. The person who started in Stage 1 and managed to push through Stage 2 is now completely exhausted mentally, emotionally and physically. There can be total collapse of body function or specific organ systems. The reserves are so depleted that the person easily becomes sick and the symptoms of disease become chronic and more degenerative. If the person continues to push forward or to suppress the symptoms, the disease process goes even deeper into the body and may finally result in failure of the whole system.

It is the relationship between the stressors and the body's stress resistance that decides when, and to what extent, ill health will result.

CHAPTER 2

The Physiology of Stress

If there is a central command post for the body's stress response it is the hypothalamus, a primitive area of the brain. The hypothalamus directly connects through an intricate array of hormonal signals to the pituitary gland and the main stress reactive glands, the adrenals. The hypothalamic-pituitary-adrenal (HPA) axis regulates heart rate, blood pressure, body temperature, sleep patterns, hunger, thirst, reproductive functions and many other body functions.

During the initial reaction to stress, there is the reaction between the hypothalamus, pituitary, the adrenal glands and the release of the main stress reactive hormones: dopamine, epinephrine (adrenalin), norepinephrine (noradrenalin) and the main stress hormone, cortisol. Even minute changes in any of these levels of hormones can have significant effects on the body and eventually on our health.

The adrenal glands are responsible for the well known fight-or-flight reaction. The hypothalamus sends out corticotropin-releasing factor (CRF) signaling the pituitary to release adrenocorticotropic hormone (ACTH) which in turn is carried in the bloodstream to the more distant adrenal glands. In response to ACTH, the production of epinephrine and cortisol is triggered, causing a sudden surge in blood sugar, heart rate and blood pressure – all the responses the body needs to flee or deal with imminent danger or crisis. These hormones under a normal stress response are carefully regulated to control everything from our immune system to our cardiovascular and behavioral systems.

THE ADRENAL GLANDS

It is interesting that many people have never heard of the adrenal glands, considering they command the most powerful hormones, which affect your body and your life. They are no bigger than a walnut and sit on top of each kidney. You cannot live without your adrenal hormones and how well you live – your quality of life – depends a great deal on how well your adrenal glands function.

The hormones secreted by your adrenals have an influence on all of the major physiological processes in your body: utilization of carbohydrates, fats and proteins; blood sugar regulation; cardiovascular and gastrointestinal functions; function of the immune system and nervous systems; inflammation and allergy reactions; and hormonal health.

Each adrenal gland consists of two parts, the cortex and the medulla. The adrenal cortex secretes a variety of steroid hormones: glucocorticoids (e.g., cortisol), mineralocorticoids (e.g., aldosterone) and androgens (e.g., testosterone). The glucocorticoids get their name from their effect on raising the level of blood sugar. The most abundant of the glucocorticoids is cortisol. Mineralocorticoids have their effect on mineral metabolism. The most important mineralocorticoid is aldosterone, which acts on the kidney promoting the reabsorption of salt into the blood to help maintain normal blood pressure. The adrenal cortex also secretes precursor hormones to androgens such as testosterone and other steroid hormones.

The inner part, adrenal medulla, makes a category of hormones called catecholamines (epinephrine and norepinephrine, previously known as adrenaline and noradrenalin). These hormones are released into the blood stream in response to physical or mental stress. Some of the effects of these neurotransmitters in the body include increased blood pressure, heart rate, blood sugar and metabolic rate. All of these effects prepare the body to take immediate and vigorous action in response to a stress (the fight-or-flight reaction.)

Adrenal fatigue or hypoadrenia is one of the most prevalent conditions in our time, yet is rarely diagnosed in Western medicine, despite being described in medical texts as far back as the 1800s. Information about non-Addison's hypoadrenia has been around for over 150 years. Today, unfortunately, this milder form of hypoadrenia is missed or misdiagnosed in doctors' offices every day, even though the patient has all of the classic symptoms.

Today, modern medicine relies strictly on clinical testing to diagnose conditions and – though clear lab testing is absolutely necessary in the diagnosis of a disease – it misses the people who may be in the earlier stages of the disease. The pre-clinical stages of a disease can have debilitating symptoms associated with it, but patients are told there is nothing wrong and that their problems are all in their head because all lab tests come back within the "normal" range. Classic examples of this are adrenal fatigue and pre-clinical hypothyroidism. The tests used to diagnose these conditions are very limiting and many people suffer unnecessarily for years. Lab tests are standardized according to statistical norms instead of the physiological optimal norms and are based on math rather than on signs and symptoms. For example – in thyroid testing, the normal range for thyroid stimulating hormone (TSH) is .4-4.2 mU/L and even though a patient may have all the classic signs of hypothyroidism and has a TSH of 3.5, most medical doctors will not treat the condition because the test has not fallen out of this standard normal range. A naturopathic doctor or holistic medical doctor will consider treating for hypothyroidism if the TSH is greater than 2.5 and the patient has the signs and symptoms of low thyroid.

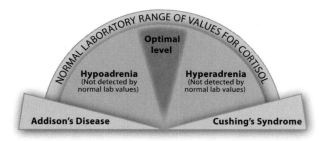

The so-called normal lab values for cortisol include all but the most extreme values. Addison's disease is at the extreme low end of adrenal function and is life threatening if left untreated. People suffering from Addison's usually need to take corticosteroid hormones for the rest of their life. This is a rare and extreme form of adrenal exhaustion and affects approximately four out of every 100,000 people.

Cushing's syndrome is at the extreme high end of adrenal function and is caused by prolonged exposure to the stress hormone cortisol. This condition, too, is relatively rare. People who are obese, have type 2 diabetes, poorly controlled blood sugar and high blood pressure have an increased risk of developing Cushing's syndrome.

ASSESSMENT OF ADRENAL FATIGUE
Standard Lab Tests
▸ *24-hour urine cortisol test* can be a helpful indicator of several adrenal steroid hormones, although the lab range considered normal is too broad to be of much value in diagnosing all but the most severe cases of hypoadrenia. (*See bell curve diagram*)
▸ *ACTH challenge test* helps evaluate the adrenal reserves and is usually only done if cortisol levels are abnormal.

There are other standard blood and urine tests used by specialists to test for adrenal disease but these tests are usually done only in the most severe cases and are beyond the scope of this book.

Saliva Adrenal Profile – Cortisol Rhythm

Saliva hormone testing measures the amounts of various stress hormones in your saliva instead of blood or urine. Saliva measures the amount of hormone inside the cells, whereas blood measures hormones outside the cells. Saliva hormone testing is beneficial in investigating the hyper and hypo adrenal states associated with dysregulation of the HPA axis. These tests are done through a naturopathic physician or complementary medical doctors.

Ragland Effect – Postural Hypotension

Normally, when a person goes from the lying position to standing, the systolic blood pressure should elevate 4-10 mm Hg (millimeters of mercury). In adrenal fatigue, the systolic blood pressure from lying to standing will either drop or stay the same. The level of drop in the blood pressure can help determine the level of adrenal fatigue.

Pupillary Response

Adrenal fatigue will cause an imbalance with sodium and potassium. One of the signs of this electrolyte imbalance is the pupillary reflex. Normally, shining a light into a person's eye will cause the pupil to constrict and it should maintain itself for 30 seconds. In the hypoadrenic person (especially in the later stages), you will find the pupil will fluctuate in size in response to the light or the pupil will initially constrict but will dilate even with continued light in less than 30 seconds.

Koenisberg Test

This is a urinary test that measures chloride and gives an indirect measurement of sodium and potassium excretion. Correlated with diet and signs and symptoms, the results of this test can be used to monitor the treatment of adrenal insufficiency. Many naturopathic doctors use this test in their clinics.

In addition, the physician needs to do a thorough history, looking at various stressful events including: surgeries and hospital stays; sicknesses such as flu, colds and pneumonia; long term pain; dental work such as root canals or implants; emotional stress such as job loss, moving, death of friend or relative, divorce, financial problems; and other stressful incidents.

A thorough patient history – coupled with the patient's signs and symptoms – is probably the most important assessment tool.

ADRENAL FATIGUE

Adrenal fatigue stretches from mild to severe forms and is caused by some form of acute severe stress or ongoing chronic stress. The stressors are varied – ranging from emotional, financial, psychological, environmental and infectious or a combination of these over a period of time. Adrenal fatigue occurs when the adrenal glands are no longer able to adequately adapt to stress.

The most common symptom (and often the first symptom seen in a hypoadrenic patient) is low energy and is more often a combination of signs and symptoms, known as a syndrome. Initially, many people with adrenal fatigue may appear quite normal but live with a feeling of always having to push themselves or use stimulants in the form of caffeine or sugar to keep them going. They may also appear lazy or unmotivated when it is really the opposite. They have to push themselves harder to merely accomplish the basic tasks. The body can only stand so much abuse and – in time – the ability to push becomes compromised. Often, the body will be telling us to rest but our mind and our will make us push ourselves. We can only do this for so long, but after awhile, when the adrenal glands become exhausted, there is nothing left to help us push on. In Western medicine these patients are treated with antipsychotic drugs for depression when really it is a physical problem – adrenal fatigue.

Common Diseases or Conditions Associated with Stress and Adrenal Fatigue

- ▶ Metabolic syndrome and diabetes
- ▶ Obesity
- ▶ Cardiovascular disease
- ▶ Anxiety disorders and depression
- ▶ Immune compromise and some cancers
- ▶ Allergies and chemical sensitivities
- ▶ Inflammatory disorders (arthritis)
- ▶ Hormonal imbalances (e.g., polycystic ovary syndrome)
- ▶ Osteoporosis
- ▶ Alzheimer's disease and memory loss
- ▶ Insomnia
- ▶ Chronic fatigue syndrome/fibromyalgia
- ▶ Asthma and bronchitis
- ▶ Gastrointestinal disorders (colitis)

There are many early symptoms that can indicate changes in the normal cortisol rhythm, reflecting pre-clinical adrenal problems. See how you score on the Adrenal Stress Indicator:

Adrenal Stress Indicator

Write the number 1 beside symptoms you have had in the past, 2 beside symptoms that occur occasionally, 3 beside symptoms that occur often, 4 beside symptoms that occur frequently. Add up the total score.

- ☐ Blurred vision/spots in front of eyes
- ☐ Hormonal imbalances (e.g., thyroid problems)
- ☐ History of asthma/bronchitis
- ☐ Prolonged exposure to stress (job, family, illness, caregiving)
- ☐ Headaches
- ☐ Environmental or chemical exposure or sensitivities
- ☐ Hypoglycemia/blood sugar problems – mood swings
- ☐ Food allergies
- ☐ Poor concentration/memory problems (Alzheimer's disease)
- ☐ Low energy, excessive fatigue
- ☐ Easily overwhelmed, inability to handle stress
- ☐ Post-exertion fatigue
- ☐ Dizziness upon standing (or fainting)
- ☐ Inflammatory conditions (arthritis, bursitis)
- ☐ Nervousness/anxiety, depression, irritability or anger
- ☐ Shortness of breath/yawning (air hunger)
- ☐ Cold hands or feet
- ☐ Low back pain, knee problems, sore muscles
- ☐ Insomnia/frequent waking
- ☐ Excessive urination
- ☐ Excessive perspiration or no perspiration
- ☐ Heart palpitations
- ☐ Edema of extremities or general edema
- ☐ Eyes light sensitive
- ☐ Cravings: sugar, salt, coffee or other stimulants
- ☐ Alcohol intolerance
- ☐ Recurrent colds or infections
- ☐ Digestive problems, ulcers
- ☐ Weight gain or weight loss
- ☐ High or low blood pressure
- ☐ Total Score

If you scored...
▶ Between 30 and 50 – you've received an early-warning indicator that your adrenals are starting to weaken
▶ Between 50 and 80 – start with adrenal support such as **AdrenaSense®**
▶ Between 80-100 – your adrenals are taxed. You may want to take an adrenal glandular product (available in health food stores) with your **AdrenaSense®**
▶ Over 100 – you are suffering from adrenal exhaustion and will require long-term adrenal support

Treatment for Adrenal Health
▶ *B-Complex* helps support the nervous system.
Suggested use: 1-2 capsules/day or as directed

▶ *Vitamin C* is very important because it is used in the formation of adrenal hormones such as cortisol. During times of stress, the body's requirement for vitamin C can increase 10 to 20 fold.
Suggested use: 2,000-4,000 mg/day (or until bowel tolerance)

▶ *Pantothenic acid* is a B vitamin and is important for energy production, helping convert glucose into energy.
Suggested use: 500 mg 3x/day

▶ *Magnesium* is important for energy production of every cell in your body and essential for adrenal gland recovery.
Suggested use: magnesium bisglycinate 200-800 mg/day
Note: magnesium may cause diarrhea even at low doses in some people, so reduce amount to your own optimal level.

▶ *GABA* (gamma-aminobutyric acid) is a neurotransmitter and works like a "brake" during times of runaway stress. Stress excites the nervous system, causing irritability, restlessness, anxiety, insomnia, seizures and movement disorders. GABA helps to regulate brain excitability.
Suggested use: 100-200 mg/day

ADAPTOGENIC HERBS FOR THE ADRENAL GLANDS

The term "adaptogen" is a category of plants that improve the response to stress. These herbs have many important properties but the most important is their normalizing effect. Regardless of the condition they help the body maintain homeostasis, the constant internal state necessary for health and life itself. For example, if the blood pressure is high, an adaptogen will help to lower it; if it is low, the same herb will help to normalize it. Some of the common health-enhancing and adrenal-supporting properties of adaptogens include:

▸ Improving blood sugar metabolism
▸ Supporting the endocrine (hormonal) system
▸ Protecting and supporting the immune system
▸ Providing liver protection and support
▸ Increasing stamina and endurance
▸ Strengthening the cardiovascular and respiratory systems
▸ Strengthening the brain and central nervous system
▸ Protecting cells from antioxidant damage

There are several adaptogenic herbs that have been studied extensively by the Russians and proven very effective in the support of the body during times of increased demands and stress. Some of the most common herbs include the herbs combined in the formula **AdrenaSense®**.

AdrenaSense – Keep It Simple

▸ ***Rhodiola rosea*** supports the cardiopulmonary system by preventing the over-release of catecholamines from the adrenals during stress. Rhodiola also supports healthy aging, energy, emotional well-being and immune system function.

▸ ***Withania somnifera*** (Ashwagandha) is considered the main adaptogen in Ayurvedic medicine. In animal studies, it supported healthy cortisol and blood sugar levels already within the normal range. Studies also found that withania supported emotional well-being and immune health.

▸ ***Siberian ginseng*** (*Eleutherococcus senticosus*) is well studied in Russian athletes and has been shown to support the body's ability to adapt to adverse physical conditions, promote mental performance, regulate heart rate and promote mental performance under stress. It is one of the most well-known adrenal adaptogens.

▸ ***Schisandra*** (*Schisandra chinensis*) is another adaptogen shown to decrease the effects of stress by supporting energy, reducing fatigue and promoting mental endurance. In combination with rhodiola and Siberian ginseng, schisandra has also been shown to help support immune function and recovery from illness.

▶ *Suma* (*Pfaffia paniculata*) has been used traditionally in Brazil for its energizing and rejuvenating effects. It provides excellent support for the cardiovascular system, central nervous system, reproductive system, digestive and immune systems.

In general, most disease conditions are caused by prolonged exposure to stress and the body's inability to continuously adapt to the stresses of life. Each person has their stress response tool box, whether it is strong genetics, a positive outlook on life or a healthy lifestyle. However, we could all benefit in today's world from reducing our stress load wherever possible and supporting the systems we rely on to help us respond to daily stressors.

By simultaneously decreasing the number and intensity of stressors in our lives and increasing our ability to handle them, we can restore our self-regulating mechanisms, prevent disease and maintain optimal health.

CHAPTER 3

Adrenal Stress and Blood Sugar Imbalances: Metabolic Syndrome, Hypoglycemia and Diabetes

HOW DOES THE BODY CONTROL BLOOD SUGAR LEVELS?

When we eat, our bodies break carbohydrates down into glucose (sugar), which is the main energy source for the body. Under normal conditions, the body maintains a very narrow range of blood glucose despite wide variations in food intake and energy demands. This balance is regulated by two hormones produced in the pancreas – insulin and glucagon – which have opposite effects. High blood glucose stimulates the secretion of insulin, which results in the cellular uptake of glucose and lowering of blood sugar.

Conversely, low levels of glucose stimulate the secretion of glucagon from the liver, which stimulates a rise in blood glucose.

The stored glucose in the liver (glycogen) is depleted fairly rapidly and when these levels are low and energy needs become high, fatty acids and amino acids are converted to glucose in the liver and kidneys (gluconeogenesis).

The adrenal glands also play an important role in blood glucose regulation. The hormone epinephrine stimulates glycogen breakdown, and cortisol promotes gluconeogenesis. Stress causes the adrenal glands to secrete more cortisol, which helps to raise blood sugars levels for more energy in response to the stressor. In turn, the increased blood sugar puts extra demands on the pancreas to secrete more insulin. When this demand on the pancreas is too great, the cells become resistance to insulin. The greater the insulin resistance, the more insulin it takes to get glucose into the cells. If stress is continuous or severe, the adrenal glands are no longer able to sustain the increase in cortisol, resulting in too little cortisol being released. This makes it difficult for the body to sustain normal levels of blood sugar.

Through the above mechanisms, the healthy body is able to maintain blood sugar levels within a narrow range, ensuring energy production in the cells. Ongoing insulin resistance and the high levels of glucose (hyperglycemia) are precursors to metabolic syndrome and type 2 diabetes.

INSULIN RESISTANCE/METABOLIC SYNDROME

One of the most common conditions in people of all ages is blood sugar dysregulation. This condition has a variety of names including hypoglycemia, insulin resistance, metabolic syndrome (syndrome X) and impaired glucose tolerance.

Blood sugar imbalances such as hypoglycemia and diabetes are well recognized and are easily diagnosed through lab tests and associated symptoms. However, in the earlier stages of insulin resistance, blood sugar imbalances are not as easily confirmed by lab tests.

In the United States, an estimated 60 to 70 million individuals are affected by insulin resistance. Statistics report that more than 40% of individuals older than 50 years may be at risk for insulin resistance; however, it can affect anyone at any age.

In order to prevent the increase in the incidence of diabetes, it is helpful to understand the important precursor to diabetes, insulin resistance or metabolic syndrome. Before a cell allows glucose in, the insulin receptor must be "turned on" by insulin. Insulin resistance occurs when the receptor has a weakened or delayed response to insulin, resulting in the inability of the cell to absorb sufficient glucose from the blood.

The primary cause of the poor insulin receptor response is the chronic over-production of insulin due to stress and/or a diet high in refined carbohydrate foods or food with a high glycemic index (GI). In order to stimulate the high glucose load, the pancreas responds by releasing abnormally high quantities of insulin. The hyperinsulinemia results in a sudden fall in blood glucose (hypoglycemia) within a couple of hours. Then, more high GI foods are ingested, causing the same thing again and again, resulting in a vicious cycle of wildly fluctuating glucose and insulin levels. If this cycle of continual bombardment of the receptors by excess insulin continues for a long period of time, this will lead to insulin resistance and an inadequate secretion of insulin by the pancreas.

Definition:
Metabolic syndrome is a group of risk factors of a metabolic origin that increase the risk of diabetes, coronary heart disease and stroke. In general, signs include abdominal obesity, dyslipidemia (high triglycerides and low HDL (good) cholesterol), elevated blood pressure and blood sugar irregularities (insulin resistance). Research shows increased levels of cortisol were found in patients with insulin resistance.

Metabolic syndrome increases the risk of type 2 diabetes anywhere from 9 to 30 times over the normal population and the risk of heart disease 2 to 4 times the normal population. It is also associated with fatty liver, kidney damage, sleep apnea, polycystic ovary syndrome (PCOS) and increased risk for dementia.

Causes:
▶ Genetic factors
▶ Insulin resistance
▶ Low grade inflammation
▶ Aging
▶ Obesity
▶ Lifestyle factors such as diet, lack of exercise, alcohol consumption

Risk Factors:
▶ Overweight, especially excess fat in the abdominal region
▶ Sedentary lifestyle
▶ Family history of type 2 diabetes, high blood pressure, cardiovascular disease
▶ History of glucose intolerance or gestational diabetes
▶ A diagnosis of elevated triglycerides/low HDL, acute pancreatitis, polycystic ovary syndrome, chronic kidney disease, cardiovascular disease

Symptoms:
In general, metabolic syndrome causes no noticeable symptoms except perhaps those related to obesity and blood sugar irregularities, which could include irritability, fatigue, fainting, dizziness, tremors, cold sweats, insomnia, anxiety, memory problems, muscle pain, night terrors, sighing and yawning, and – in rare instances – convulsions.

Diagnosis:
A thorough medical history and physical exam along with lab tests should be done if you suspect metabolic syndrome. Early detection is very important in preventing the more chronic diseases associated with metabolic syndrome.

Lab Tests for Diabetes and Metabolic Syndrome May Include:
▸ Fasting blood sugar (FBS) and a post-meal two- and four-hour glucose challenge or a two-hour glucose challenge
▸ Fasting insulin
▸ Lipid panel: HDL, LDL, triglycerides, total cholesterol
▸ Increased cortisol levels (stress)
▸ Other tests should include blood pressure and calculation of body mass index (BMI) and waist circumference
▸ A blood pressure of 130/85 or more and a waist circumference greater than 40 inches in Caucasian men (35 inches in Asian men) or 35 inches in Caucasian women (31 in Asian women) can be indicative of metabolic syndrome

CALCULATING BODY MASS INDEX
BMI in pounds (weight in pounds divided by [height in inches x height in inches] multiplied by 703)
Example: 120 lbs divided by (65" x 65" = 4225) multiplied by 703 = 19.96

BMI

$$\frac{\text{(Weight in pounds)}}{\text{(Height in inches x height in inches)}} \times 703 = \text{BMI}$$

BMI in Kilograms

$$\frac{\text{(Weight in kilograms)}}{\text{(Height in meters x height in meters)}} = \text{BMI}$$

WEIGHT STATUS	BMI
Underweight	Below 18.5
Normal	18.5-24.9
Overweight	25.0-29.9
Obese	30.0 and above

Obesity has been defined as a BMI ≥ 30.0 in World Health Organization (WHO) classification but it does not take into account the morbidity and mortality associated with milder degrees of overweight. A significant increase in risk of death from cardiovascular disease was found for all BMIs of > 25.0 in women and 26.5 in men. There is a direct relationship between a BMI up to 30.0 and the relative risk of several chronic conditions caused by excess body fat such as type 2 diabetes, hypertension, coronary artery disease and gallstones.

Nutritional and dietary treatment of metabolic syndrome and type 2 diabetes are very similar. Please refer to treatment after the next section on diabetes for nutritional recommendations.

Treatment of the Underlying Causes

- ▶ Reduce excess weight by at least 10% in the next 6-12 months
- ▶ Increase physical activity to 30 to 60 minutes of moderate aerobic exercise at least four days per week
- ▶ Decrease blood pressure to below 130/85 mmHg with diet, exercise and stress reduction
- ▶ Reduce triglycerides and improve HDL through diet, exercise and supplementation with essential fatty acids (e.g., omega-3)
- ▶ "Society of Sitters" = health hazard

The average adult spends over 90% of his or her waking hours sitting. This "Society of Sitters" go from the breakfast table, to the car, to the desk, back to the table and then to the couch to read or watch TV. Only 1-5% of waking hours are spent performing moderate to physical activity with only 0.5% of this activity being sustained for at least 10 minutes. It has been found that each 2-hour increase in sitting time is associated with a 5-23% increase in the risk of obesity and 7-14% increase in the risk of type 2 diabetes, as well as an increased probability of metabolic syndrome and ovarian cancer. According to a study published in the July 2009 edition of the Current Cardiovascular Risk Results, prolonged sitting is a "health hazard." So, how do you conquer the negative effects of prolonged sitting when you have a desk job? Yes, exercise helps, but it is only part of the solution. Researchers evaluated the health of men and women who reported exercising 5 days a week for 30 minutes, a standard that is considered active enough to have health benefits. The results were surprising — waist size, blood pressure and cholesterol levels were still all negatively affected by the amount of time spent sitting and these results were more pronounced in women than in men. The researchers labeled the people who sit all day but still find time to exercise "active couch potatoes." So, what can you do if regular exercise doesn't counteract the ill effects of sitting?

Get up and move! Often!

Simple activities like standing to answer the phone, getting up to fill your water glass, taking the stairs ….. walking and moving whenever you can. Researchers found that people who took frequent breaks during long periods of sedentary activity had a waist circumference that, on average, was 2 inches less than that of people who did not get out of their chair.

Start kicking the sitting habit now and take five minutes of every hour to get out of your chair and stretch, stand or walk.

Obesity and Overweight

According to the American Heart and Stroke Foundation 2013, among Americans 20 years old and older, 154.7 million are overweight or obese (BMI of 25.0 and higher). Of these, 78.4 million are obese (BMI of 30.0 and higher). The obesity epidemic in children age 12-19 continues to grow: 24.9 million are overweight and 12.8 million of these are obese. With smoking rates declining and obesity escalating, obesity is now an equal if not greater threat than smoking to the shortening of life. As previously mentioned, overweight and obese people are at a much greater risk for metabolic syndrome, diabetes and heart disease.

Why Stress Can Make You Fat

In a stressful situation, your adrenals put out increased levels of cortisol, norepinephrine and epinephrine to give more energy for the stressful event. Cortisol increases fat deposition, especially around the belly.

ADRENAL FATIGUE AND HYPOGLYCEMIA

Hypoglycemia is diagnosed when blood glucose falls to abnormally low levels due to imbalances in the hormones that regulate blood sugar.

Hypoglycemia commonly occurs during adrenal fatigue when low levels of the adrenal hormones epinephrine, norepinephrine and cortisol are combined with the high insulin levels of stress. Glucose levels fail to rise enough to meet the increased energy demands and as a result the cells do not get the glucose they require and experience some of the symptoms of hypoglycemia. The liver's role in the regulation of glucose was discussed earlier in this section.

Further complicating the matter is the higher insulin levels. Insulin opens the cell wall membranes so the cells can take in more glucose for fuel. Cortisol helps to regulate the amount of glucose getting to the cells, thereby protecting the cells from the effects of too much glucose and the body from too rapid a decline in blood sugar. When cortisol levels are lowered due to adrenal fatigue, this balancing process is less regulated. In the presence of the increased insulin and decreased adrenal hormones, blood sugar levels drop rapidly.

Hypoglycemia can be divided broadly into three categories: reactive, drug induced and fasting.

Reactive hypoglycemia is a term describing hypoglycemia symptoms that occur two to four hours after eating (postprandial). It is thought to be a consequence of increased absorption of glucose from the small intestine and excessive insulin is triggered by a meal high in carbohydrates. The causes of reactive hypoglycemia are often unknown but can be related to increased sensitivity to epinephrine, an adrenal stress hormone released during times of stress or a deficiency in glucagon release. Reactive hypoglycemia is often ignored or overlooked because it is harder to diagnose, as low glucose levels are not always found at the time of testing.

Drug Induced Hypoglycemia

Drugs used in the treatment of diabetes are used to lower blood glucose levels. When used in excess, blood glucose levels drop too rapidly, leading to hypoglycemia.

Fasting Hypoglycemia

Fasting hypoglycemia occurs after strenuous exercise or during an extended period between meals. It occurs commonly in people who drink alcohol heavily or have liver disease or adrenal fatigue.

Hypoglycemia may be caused by tumors, autoimmune disorders, kidney and liver disease or hormonal disorders.

Symptoms of Hypoglycemia and Insulin Resistance

The symptoms may vary from person to person, but will include the following: sweating, shakiness, heart palpitations, irritability, anxiety due to secretion of adrenal hormones, weakness and tiredness, dizziness or fainting, difficulty concentrating, confusion, blurred vision, seizure, loss of consciousness, and in extreme cases coma and death. If hypoglycemia is suspected, blood glucose levels are measured. See tests for metabolic syndrome.

Many people who have had hypoglycemia for years are at greater risk for developing diabetes due to the added demands on the pancreatic and adrenal hormones.

Follow the dietary and lifestyle recommendations in the diabetes section below:

DIABETES

Based on data from the National Diabetes Fact Sheet 2011, there are 25.8 million children and adults living with diabetes in the U.S. and 79 million people with prediabetes. The World Health Organization predicts that by the year 2025, 300 million people worldwide will have diabetes.

Rising obesity rates, an aging population and changes in the ethnic mix of new immigrants are believed to be driving the increasing rates of diabetes. Diabetes rates are 18% higher among people from South Asia, 66% higher among people of Hispanic descent and 77% higher among African Americans.

Total health care and related costs for the treatment of diabetes is estimated to be $174 billion annually.

Diabetes is a condition in which the body cannot properly store or use fuel for energy. To utilize glucose, the body's main fuel source, insulin, is required. Insulin is made by the pancreas and allows glucose to leave the blood and enter the cells for energy. Diabetes develops when the pancreas cannot make enough insulin or when the cells become resistant and do not respond to insulin, resulting in high levels of glucose in the blood. There are three main types of diabetes. **Type 1** diabetes, previously known as insulin dependent diabetes mellitus (IDDM) or juvenile diabetes, typically strikes before the age of 30. The pancreas is not able to produce insulin and the immune system or environmental factors are believed to trigger Type 1 which accounts for 5-10% of diabetes. **Type 2** diabetes is the most common and is discussed at more length below. Previously known as noninsulin-dependent diabetes mellitus (NIDDM) or adult onset diabetes, type 2 diabetes affects over 90% of people with diabetes. About 70% of people over age 70 have type 2 diabetes. **Type 3** diabetes is gestational diabetes and affects 2-5% of pregnancies. Those who develop gestational diabetes have a greater risk of developing diabetes later in life.

Risk Factors for Type 2 Diabetes

▸ Advanced age
▸ Being overweight
▸ Family history of diabetes
▸ Developed gestational diabetes during pregnancy
▸ Having high blood pressure and/or high cholesterol
▸ High refined carbohydrate diet
▸ Sedentary lifestyle

Signs and Symptoms of Diabetes

▸ Unquenchable thirst
▸ Frequent urination
▸ Weight changes (gain or loss)
▸ Fatigue or lack of energy especially after eating
▸ Blurred vision
▸ Frequent bladder or yeast infections
▸ Male impotence (erectile dysfunction)
▸ Slow healing of cuts or sores

People with diabetes are at a greater risk for problems that involve damage to the small blood vessels and nerves and for the development of hardening of the arteries (atherosclerosis), which can result in heart attacks, strokes and poor blood flow to extremities and the brain (vascular dementia). Damage to the small blood vessels affects the eyes, specifically the retina. This is called diabetic retinopathy and is the leading cause of blindness. Damage to the kidneys – called diabetic nephropathy – leads to kidney failure and the need for dialysis. Damage to the nerves that supply the arms, legs and gastrointestinal tract is called neuropathy. Peripheral neuropathy has poor blood flow and the legs may eventually need to be amputated.

As you can see, this is not a pretty picture and what makes it more difficult to accept is that diabetes, in most cases, is preventable through diet and exercise.

Diagnosing Type 2 Diabetes

Your doctor will take a medical history and run some blood and urine lab tests (see metabolic syndrome). A common finding in the diagnosis of diabetes is protein and sugar in the urine. Increased fasting glucose and elevated triglycerides are also common. If the fasting blood glucose level is 126 mg/dL or higher, a diagnosis of diabetes is made. If the fasting blood glucose level is between 110-125 mg/dL, the person has as a higher risk for diabetes down the road. However, many people are in the prediabetic state and blood sugar levels will still be in the "normal" ranges.

The main goal of diabetes management is to maintain blood glucose levels within the normal range. Weight control, diet and exercise are extremely important. The most important control of diabetes is nutritional.

Diet and Lifestyle for Metabolic Syndrome and Diabetes

▶ Limit foods with high sugar content, especially on an empty stomach. Refer to glycemic index sources and keep 80-90% of food intake in the low to moderate glycemic index range.

▶ Eliminate as much as possible refined carbohydrates (white breads, pastas, pizza, desserts, soda pop, etc.)

▶ Eat small frequent meals and snacks high in protein

▶ Eat a diet high in fiber, fresh vegetables and fruits, good quality protein and good oils such as flax and olive oil

▶ Carry some juice or dried fruit for when you feel your blood sugar drop

▶ Exercise is a very important aspect of a healthy lifestyle to both prevent and help with the treatment of blood sugar problems such as insulin resistance and diabetes

▶ If you are overweight, find a program that can help you lose weight. Losing even 5 to 10 lbs can help regulate blood glucose levels

Prevention of any disease is the number one goal and the best thing for prevention of metabolic syndrome and diabetes is a good diet and exercise.

Nutritional Supplements for Healthy Blood Sugar Support
▶ *Chromium* is considered one of the most important nutrients for regulating blood sugar. It has been shown to augment the action of insulin, thereby reducing insulin requirements in those taking insulin.
Suggested use: 200-400 mcg/day

▶ *Magnesium* is profoundly affected by stress. It is important for energy production and blood sugar control.
Suggested use: 100-400 mg/day

▶ *Zinc* is important for the production of insulin.
Suggested use: 30-60 mg/day

▶ *B vitamins* are depleted by stress. A deficiency in B6 in particular can contribute to blood sugar problems.
Suggested use: 1-2 capsules/day of a B complex or as directed on bottle

Digestive health is important in the treatment of blood sugar irregularities. Seventy percent of the body's immune system is located in the gut. Cytokines in the gut can blunt the insulin response. The factors that create excessive production of cytokines include food sensitivities, candidiasis and parasites. All of these can be caused by poor diet, overuse of antibiotics, immune suppressing medications and STRESS.

▶ *Ultimate Probiotic* helps support healthy gut flora.
Suggested use: 1 capsule 3x/day

▶ *AdrenaSense*® supports healthy blood sugar levels already within the normal range. AdrenaSense helps regulates stress hormones.
Suggested use: 2 capsules midday with food

▶ *PGX*® (*PolyGlycopleX*®) is a super fiber complex made up of 100% natural, highly viscous polysaccharides (plant fibers). PGX expands in the stomach creating a feeling of fullness by absorbing water and filling the stomach. This slows digestion and the absorption of carbohydrates, effectively lowering the glycemic index of the food and supporting a lower, more stable blood sugar response which also helps manage cravings. PGX supports healthy weight loss, supports healthy blood sugar and cholesterol levels already within the normal range, reduces food cravings and lowers the glycemic index of food, beverage or meal.

For further information on PGX please visit www.pgx.com.

▶ *Cinnamon* is a potent inducer of insulin sensitivity and as little as one gram a day can reduce blood sugar levels by up to 30%. It enhances enzymes that increase insulin receptor sensitivity and inhibits those with the opposite action. It also lowers lipid levels and reduces oxidative stress.

▶ *Vitamin D* – both type 1 and type 2 diabetes are profoundly linked to low vitamin D levels.
Suggested use: 1,000-2,000 IU/day

For many people, following a healthy diet and exercise program may be all that is required to help control glucose levels. For others, this may not be enough to lower glucose levels and they may need to take medications in order to sustain glucose in a normal range.

Medications for type 2 diabetes are taken by mouth or injection. There are several types of oral diabetes medications, so talk to your doctor about what medication would be best for you.

CHAPTER 4

Adrenal Stress and Cardiovascular Disease

According to the World Health Organization (WHO), it is estimated that 30% of all deaths globally each year (approximately 18 million people) are from cardiovascular disease.

Heart disease and stroke are the leading causes of death in the U.S. and pose a significant threat to millions of others, according to the American Heart Association's Heart Disease and Stroke Statistical Update.

▶ More than 787,000 people in the U.S. died from heart disease, stroke and other cardiovascular diseases in 2010. That's about one of every three deaths in America

▶ Cardiovascular diseases claim more lives than all forms of cancer combined

▶ About 83.6 million Americans are living with some form of cardiovascular disease or the after-effects of stroke

▶ Someone in the U.S. dies from heart disease about every 90 seconds

Direct and indirect costs of cardiovascular diseases and stroke total more than $315.4 billion. That includes health expenditures and lost productivity. Very ALARMING!

In an era of high-tech medicinal wonders, medical researchers have recently found a free and easy way to predict a woman's risk of future heart attack: take her pulse.

It was found that those women with the highest resting pulse – more than 76 beats per minute – were more likely to suffer a heart attack or die from coronary heart disease than women with the lowest resting pulse – 62 beats per minute or less. Doctors have known for years that heart rate predicts heart attack risk in men and the higher a man's resting pulse the greater the risk, but until recently, there was no good evidence that the same held true for women.

As previously mentioned, metabolic syndrome and type 2 diabetes are common risk factors for cardiovascular disease. A reduction in insulin sensitivity can cause elevated triglycerides (TG) and lowered HDL (good) cholesterol. These changes can be predictive of cardiovascular disease.

The overall cholesterol level is not important. More crucial is the level of LDL (bad cholesterol) as it can be a troublemaker — too much of it can lead to atherosclerosis, angina, heart attacks and strokes. HDL is the garbage collector that collects waste materials including excess LDL and carries the garbage back to the liver for processing. Higher levels of HDL are beneficial.

Cholesterol is transported through the bloodstream by lipoproteins and there are two types that carry most of the cholesterol: low-density-lipoprotein (LDL) and high-density-lipoprotein (HDL). Both HDL and LDL have different functions in your body and in balance are not bad or good.

HIGH CHOLESTEROL DOES NOT CAUSE HEART DISEASE

Most people and some doctors still believe that excess cholesterol in the blood can lead to angina, heart attacks and strokes. But what is unreported is that not all cholesterol is harmful. In fact, cholesterol plays a vital role in our health. Cholesterol is an essential component in our cell membranes, acts as an antioxidant, is used in brain/nerve communication and repairs lesions in the membranes of arteries and veins. Cholesterol also acts as a precursor for the synthesis of vitamins D, E and K; for the production of steroid hormones such as cortisol, estrogen, progesterone and testosterone; and for calcitriol which regulates calcium.

It is not the cholesterol levels or the cholesterol-containing foods that are the culprits in heart disease. Cholesterol has been blamed because upon inspection of the arteries of someone who has had, or is at risk for, a heart attack the levels of plaque containing cholesterol are very high.

Inflammation in the body can be caused by ongoing stress, poor dietary habits and a deficiency of antioxidants, to name a few. The inflammation causes damage to the lining of the blood vessels, and cholesterol is transported to the tissues as part of the inflammatory response to repair the damage. It will only lodge itself onto the artery and cause plaque buildup if the artery has become damaged. Cholesterol is not the bad guy and it is becoming a well-known fact that the main cause of coronary artery disease is chronic inflammation.

Atherosclerosis is characterized by chronic inflammation involving the immune system response. So, a more important question to ask is how do we prevent and decrease the amount of inflammation in our bodies, rather than how can we reduce cholesterol-containing foods and cholesterol levels?

EFFECTS OF STRESS ON ATHEROSCLEROSIS AND CARDIOVASCULAR DISEASE

Adrenal stress hormones, glucocorticoids, are powerful anti-inflammatory agents, but in chronic stress, a problem can occur in the feedback loop of the HPA axis and as a result the fight-or-flight response remains active. Eventually this causes cells in the immune system to release cytokines, which are molecules that promote inflammation.

The effects of stress can cause abnormalities in the biofeedback loop of the HPA axis, which causes a pro-inflammatory response.

Abnormalities in the HPA axis have been described in several chronic inflammatory disorders. It is clear that stress can create significant damage to the cardiovascular system by elevating blood pressure and increasing the risk of coronary artery disease, atherosclerosis and heart attack.

Stress also causes the blood to become thicker, and the combination of a narrowing of the arteries due to plaque and blood sludge put considerable stress on the heart and blood vessels. Due to the narrowing of arteries and blood thickening, blood pressure increases and plaque is often dislodged and travels in the bloodstream and becomes a ticking time bomb. If it gets stuck in one of the heart arteries, it triggers a heart attack or if trapped in a blood vessel in the brain, can cause a stroke.

EMOTIONAL STRESS

The heart is smooth muscle, but recent research has discovered a "neuronal sheath" strikingly similar to the neocortical neurons of the brain. The heart, as considered by many traditional cultures, may indeed be the seat of the human spirit. Research on the scientific mechanism of the age-old wisdom that it is possible to die of a "broken heart" is being done and so far, it is safe to say that scientists are finding that depression is an independent risk factor for the development of both coronary artery disease and stroke.

Stress and the emotions associated with stress are important risk factors for cardiovascular disease. The Mayo Clinic reported that among individuals with existing coronary artery disease, the strongest predictor of future cardiac events is psychological health. When researchers interviewed heart attack survivors, they found the intensity and timing of stressful emotions like anger, anxiety and worry dramatically increased their risk.

There is more and more medical literature on the effects of negative emotions such as anxiety, fear, depression and anger on cardiovascular disease. Add to these the effects of chronic stressors such as job stress, difficult relationships, financial problems, the burden of caregiving or living in chronic pain. The adverse cardiovascular effects can be severe or even fatal.

EFFECTS OF CHRONIC STRESS ON THE CARDIOVASCULAR AND METABOLIC SYSTEMS

Scientific research indicates chronic stress can:

▶ increase risk of coronary heart disease – increase risk of tachycardia, atrial or ventricular fibrillation – elevate blood pressure and heart rate

▶ increase atherosclerosis – increase the risk of myocardial infarction (heart attack) – increase the risk of diabetes – increase the likelihood of obesity

Reference: McEwen BS. Protective and damaging effects of stress mediators. *New England Journal of Medicine*. 1998;338(3):171-179

Other causes of atherosclerosis include diets high in hydrogenated oils. Hydrogenation involves saturating an oil with hydrogen atoms and heating it as high as 384°F. This process turns the oil into a solid. The molecular structure changes to the extent that it becomes unrecognizable by the body, a trans fatty acid. These trans fats are found in margarines, baked goods, some ice creams and most snack foods like potato chips, corn chips, etc. In the refining of other oils, temperatures up to 482°F are used which causes nutrient destruction and trans fatty acids.

For optimal health, choose expeller pressed unprocessed extra virgin olive oil, flax oil, sesame oil and fish oil.

If oils are dangerous when heated, how can we safely cook with them? Some oils offer more heat stability than others. Use sesame oil, olive oil, cocoa butter or butter when cooking at LOW heats. If oil becomes black or brown during cooking, discard it.

The researchers for the Framingham Heart Study, somewhat of a gold standard for the prediction of heart disease, concluded that cholesterol was a risk factor for heart disease. However, if you look at the study you will see that half the people with heart disease had low cholesterol and half the people without heart disease had high cholesterol. Most studies found that for women, high cholesterol is NOT a risk factor for heart disease. A Canadian study that followed 5,000 healthy middle-aged men for 12 years found that high cholesterol was not associated with heart disease. Another study done at the University of Toronto revealed the following: men with low cholesterol were just as susceptible to a second heart attack as men with high cholesterol.

In Russia, studies show that it is those with lower cholesterol that have higher incidence of heart disease. The hypothesis of coronary heart disease as the result of excessive intake of saturated fats may no longer be sustainable.

These are small sample studies that contradict the idea that cholesterol is the bad guy in heart disease. So why has this misinformation held "true" for so long?

Perhaps one of the reasons is that the statin drugs (Lipitor, Zocor, Mevacor, etc.) are major money makers and they definitely do lower cholesterol levels. But if cholesterol is not directly associated with risk of heart disease, why are these drugs necessary?

Statin drugs block a vital step in the synthesis of cholesterol and as a result, the synthesis of coenzyme Q10 (ubiquinone) and squalene, both precursors to cholesterol, are also blocked. Coenzyme Q10 (CoQ10) is very important for healthy heart function and, coupled with vitamin E, is important for energy metabolism in muscles. This is why muscle pain is such a common side effect of statin drugs. CoQ10 is also important for healthy brain function and when decreased through the use of statin drugs or otherwise, memory is affected. Squalene is an antioxidant and a potent fighter of cancer cells. If you are going to continue to take your statin drugs, supplementing with CoQ10 and squalene may be helpful.

I realize that suggesting that cholesterol levels are not associated with heart disease flies in the face of current dogma. However, from all of the information I have seen, it appears that keeping the triglycerides lower and HDL higher are more important than recommending drugs or natural remedies to lower overall cholesterol. A diet high in healthy fats and low in refined carbohydrates and sugars most often can maintain healthy TG and HDL levels.

If we all ate saturated fat and cholesterol in the form of animal fats, eggs and full-fat dairy and were heart disease-free until the early 1900s, what changed?

When we started replacing these foods with processed heated oils, sugar and refined foods, heart disease rates started to climb. Cholesterol and saturated fats stand wrongly accused. As the incidence of heart disease has increased, so too have the stress demands and the continued addiction to fast foods due to never having time during the day to pay attention to healthy eating. If you don't believe any of this and if you are taking or considering taking cholesterol lowering drugs, please review the following information before making a decision: *The Cholesterol Myths: Exposing the Fallacy that Saturated Fat and Cholesterol Cause Heart Disease by Dr. U. Ravnskov, MD, PhD; Know Your Fats: The Complete Primer for Understanding the Nutrition of Fats, Oils and Cholesterol by Mary Enig; and The Schwarzbein Principle by Dr. D. Schwarzbein, MD.*

TESTS THAT MAY PREDICT RISK FOR HEART DISEASE
The Conventional Cholesterol Model

As mentioned previously, the accepted culprit in this model is the low-density-lipoprotein (LDL) that transports cholesterol and triglycerides from the liver to the peripheral tissues. The high-density-lipoprotein (HDL) exhibits protective effects by transporting the free cholesterol back to the liver for excretion.

▸ *Triglycerides* – insulin resistance can cause high triglycerides, which can be a risk factor for heart disease
▸ *LDL/HDL ratio* – it is important to maintain a higher level of HDL
▸ *Apolipoprotein B (apoB)* – apoB is the primary apolipoprotein of the low-density-lipoproteins (LDL or bad cholesterol) and is responsible for carrying cholesterol to the tissues. High levels of apoB can lead to plaque that cause vascular disease (atherosclerosis) and has been found to be a better predictor of heart disease than LDL.
▸ *Lipoprotein (a)* – is a strong risk factor for coronary artery disease, cerebrovascular disease, atherosclerosis, thrombosis and stroke. Lipoprotein (a) levels are only slightly affected by diet, exercise and other environmental factors and commonly prescribed lipid-reducing drugs have little or no effect. Similar to LDL, high Lp(a) predicts the risk of early atherosclerosis but in advanced atherosclerosis, Lp(a) is an independent risk factor not dependent on LDL. In cases of elevated Lp(a), Aspirin has been shown to lower levels up to 80%.
▸ *C-reactive protein (CRP)* – a general marker for infection and inflammation. Ask for the high-sensitivity CRP (hs-CRP) test.
▸ *Homocysteine* – a common amino acid related to early development of heart and blood vessel disease. In fact, it is considered an independent risk factor for heart disease. And even slightly elevated levels can significantly increase risk.
▸ *Salivary cortisol* – assessment of stress hormone levels throughout the day
▸ *Pulse* – a pulse rate of more than 76 beats per minute represents a higher risk for heart disease
▸ *Blood pressure* – high blood pressure increases the risk of coronary artery disease

Heart disease is often called the "silent killer" because all tests may be in the normal range and many people have few or no symptoms and do not even know that they have it.

Hair Gives a Heads-Up on Heart Attack Risk

A new study published in the journal *Stress* found that the **stress hormone cortisol** can be measured in hair, providing the first long-term record of chronic stress. In this study high levels of cortisol in the hair were associated with heart attacks. This test may be used to identify people at risk for cardiovascular disease.

Risk Factors for Heart Disease

▶ *Increasing age* – over 83% of people who die of coronary heart disease are 65 or older

▶ *Heredity and race* – children of parents with heart disease are more likely to develop it themselves. African-Americans, Mexican-Americans and First Nations people are at higher risk, partly due to higher rates of obesity and diabetes.

▶ *Smoking* – smokers' risk of developing coronary heart disease is two to four times that of non-smokers

▶ *Cholesterol* – discussed earlier. It is important to maintain a high level of HDL and a low level of triglycerides.

▶ *High blood pressure* – indicates the heart's workload, causing the heart to thicken and become stiffer

▶ *Physical inactivity* – regular moderate exercise helps prevent heart disease

▶ *Obesity and overweight* – people who have excess body fat are more likely to develop heart disease and stroke even if they have no other risk factors

▶ *Diabetes and metabolic syndrome* – significantly increases the risk of developing heart disease

▶ *Stress* and the inflammatory response caused by increased stress hormones are known to be a significant risks for heart disease

▶ *Excess alcohol* – can cause increased blood pressure, contribute to elevated triglycerides and increase risk of obesity and heart disease as well as many other alcohol related diseases. The risk of heart disease in moderate drinkers (one drink for women, two for men per day) was lower than in non-drinkers.

▶ *Young adults* are the new at-risk group for heart disease in Canada.

Supplement Suggestions for Supporting Heart Health

▶ *AdrenaSense®* helps regulate stress hormones.
  Suggested use: 2 capsules midday with food
  Note: Siberian ginseng, an adaptogenic herb found in AdrenaSense, helps support healthy blood pressure levels already within the normal range.

Panax ginseng, on the other hand, has been known to elevate blood pressure in some people.

▶ *Coenzyme Q10* – Heart tissue biopsies in patients with various heart conditions have a CoQ10 deficiency in 50-75% of the cases. Many studies show its effectiveness in the treatment of high blood pressure, atherosclerosis, angina, congestive heart failure and cardio-myopathy. It seems to work better when taken with vitamin E.
Note: Be aware that medications for hypertension and high cholesterol deplete CoQ10.
Suggested use: 50-150 mg/day or 2 mg for each kg of body weight. Some experts say the sicker the cardiac patient, the higher the CoQ10 levels need to be.

▶ *Essential fatty acids* help support healthy inflammatory responses and healthy arteries. They can be added to the diet in the form of flax oil, pumpkin seed oil or mixed blends containing omega-3 and omega-6 fatty acids. Some people prefer fish oils in the form of capsules.
Suggested use: Rx Omega-3 2 softgels 1-3x/day

▶ *Calcium* regulation is vital to the normal contraction and relaxation of the heart muscle. Oxidative stress (free radical damage) is a common cause of heart disease in many people as it causes the regulation of calcium to become unbalanced.
Suggested use: 600-800 mg/day

▶ *Vitamin C* with bioflavonoids is well known as an antioxidant that prevents oxidation of LDL, raises HDL and lowers triglycerides. Vitamin C is an essential part of any health program and may help prevent atherosclerosis.
Suggested use: 1,500-2,000 mg/day

▶ *Magnesium* – is essential for normal heart muscle function and can alleviate arrhythmias and heart palpitations.
Suggested use: 200-400 mg/day

▶ *Proanthocyanidins* (PACs) are a class of antioxidants found in foods such as grape seeds, barley, chocolate, red wine, rose hips, apples and berries. PACs have been shown to help prevent cardiovascular disease, improve blood circulation and reduce platelet aggregation, a common cause of stroke. Grape seed extract is available in supplement form and is a good source of PACs.
Suggested use: 100 mg 2x/day

▸ *Garlic* improves circulation and has been shown to reduce blood pressure. Use liberally in foods or take as a supplement.
Suggested use: 1,000-3,000 mg/day

▸ *Vitamin E* mixed tocopherols is an antioxidant that improves blood flow and reduces fatty plaques.
Note: Do not take with blood thinners such as Warfarin.
Suggested use: 200-400 IU/day

▸ *Lipoic acid* is a powerful antioxidant that prevents free radical formation thereby protecting the cardiovascular system. It is both fat and water soluble, easily transported to all tissues and cells of the body and able to cross the blood-brain barrier. Lipoic acid protects against LDL oxidation and reduces inflammation thereby helping to prevent atherosclerosis and other cardiovascular disease.
Suggested use: 50-150 mg/day (up to 500 mg/day can be taken without side effects)

▸ *Vitamin D* – Most people suffering from atherosclerosis and heart disease are chronically deficient in vitamin D. There is a strong inverse relationship between vitamin D levels and artery calcification; the more D in the blood, the less calcification. Artery cells have vitamin D receptors (VDR) which, when stimulated by vitamin D, inhibit the deposit of calcium.
Suggested use: 1,000-3,000 IU/day

▸ *Cholesterol Formula* combines plant sterols with Sytrinol® for a comprehensive formula that promotes heart health and supports healthy cholesterol levels already within the normal range. This formula also supports healthy inflammatory responses, further supporting heart health.
Suggested use: 2 capsules 2x/day

▸ *Multivitamin and mineral* helps ensure adequate intake of nutrients and the B vitamins help with stress as well as provide other essential support.
Suggested use: as directed

The effects of olive oil on coronary heart disease (CHD) and hypertension epidemiological studies demonstrate that the Mediterranean diet reduces the incidence of CHD. The antioxidant effects of olive oil may contribute to these protective effects by preventing the oxidation of LDL. There is also a reduced incidence of hypertension in populations that follow the Mediterranean diet.

Several studies have demonstrated the antihypertensive properties of olive oil. It is suggested that the mechanism for blood pressure reduction is that olive oil is a calcium channel antagonist closely related to the common calcium channel blocker drugs.

There are several interesting studies showing the positive effects of meditation for the management of stress related disorders such as hypertension and other risk factors for heart disease. The physiological effects of meditation include decreased heart rate, reduced respiratory rate, reduced blood pressure, lower cortisol levels and reduced free radicals.

Other Health Tips to Decrease Your Risk Factors for Cardiovascular Disease

▸ *Exercise* – a lack of exercise has been found to be a primary factor in reducing the risk of heart disease, diabetes and obesity. Even walking 30 minutes 3 times a week decreases your risk of heart attack by 30%. Gentle jogging or increasing walking speed can reduce risk up to 60%. A recent study published in the *Journal of the American Medical Association* found that leisure time and physical activity decreased heart disease by 50%.

▸ *Water, water, water* – keeping well hydrated can help maintain healthy blood flow. As little as five or six glasses of water daily can cut your risk of heart disease in half.

▸ *Quit smoking*

▸ *Diet* – a diet high in fruits and vegetables, fish (a good source of essential fatty acids) and lean meats (i.e., Mediterranean diet) can considerably reduce the risk of heart disease as well as other chronic disease.

▸ *Rest and relaxation* – make sure you get adequate sleep and find ways to reduce your stress, such as exercise or meditation. Sleep deprivation increases the risk of obesity, diabetes and hypertension.

▸ *Eliminate refined carbohydrates* – refined carbohydrates stimulate the release of insulin, which has many harmful effects in the body. Through a series of steps in the body, high insulin levels promote fat storage, increase blood pressure, shut off fat-burning pathways and turn on pathways that produce fat and triglycerides. Arterial damage and plaque formation (atherosclerosis) is also increased.

▶ *Emotional state* – don't worry, be happy – studies at Harvard Medical School show that negative emotions such as anger, depression, worry or anxiety are linked to an increased risk for heart disease. In older adults, it has been found that depression is associated with a greater than 50% risk of heart failure.

▶ *Consumption of fats and oils* – Don't get caught up in the "fat phobia." Good fats do not promote heart disease or cholesterol problems. Instead of hydrogenated and heated oils – such as margarines, deep fried foods and processed oils – use essential fatty acids (omega-3 and omega-6) from flax, pumpkin seed and fish oils. Olive oil is also good for the heart. Animal fats are not the bad guys – heated, refined oils are.

CHAPTER 5

Adrenal Stress and Menopause

Menopause represents a major transition period in the lives of most women. Most women enter menopause between the ages of 45 and 55. The definition of menopause is one year with no menstrual cycle. On average, 70-80% of women will experience mild to moderate symptoms, while 10-15% will suffer severe symptoms. Some of the most common symptoms include anxiety, hot flashes, night sweats, sleep problems, brain fog and memory problems, mood swings, irritability, depression, weight gain, urinary incontinence, recurring urinary or vaginal infections, and fatigue.

During this time, women experience a decreased production of sex hormones by the ovaries and the adrenal glands and fat cells take over. Then, the liver packages the hormones and the thyroid also plays a role. When the adrenal glands are constantly having to adapt to a stress, progesterone is converted to the adrenal stress hormones such as cortisol, rather than converting to estrogens and testosterone in the steroid pathway.

So, you can see menopause is much more than the ovaries going on a well-deserved vacation. Whether or not the hormonal transition will be symptomatic or relatively symptom free depends on the health of these organs. Women with a congested liver, adrenal fatigue or thyroid problems will have a much more difficult time during menopause.

The adrenal-thyroid feedback interaction is very important as many women not only have adrenal fatigue entering into menopause but also clinical or pre-clinical hypothyroid function.

ADRENAL-THYROID RELATIONSHIP
One of cortisol's more important functions is to act in concert with thyroid

hormones. Cortisol makes the thyroid work more efficiently – not too low and not too high. It is very important for normal thyroid function and this is why many people who have an imbalance in adrenal cortisol levels usually have thyroid symptoms. Both cortisol and thyroid hormones have to be in the cells, bound to their respective receptors for optimal thyroid function. When cortisol levels are low, caused by adrenal exhaustion, the thyroid is less efficient at doing its job.

When cortisol levels get too high, again due to the adrenal response to stressors, it causes the tissues to no longer respond to the thyroid hormone signal. It creates a condition of thyroid resistance, meaning that the thyroid hormone levels may be normal but the tissues fail to respond to the thyroid signal. This resistance to the thyroid hormone caused by elevated cortisol levels applies also to all other hormones such as insulin, progesterone, estrogens, testosterone and cortisol itself. When cortisol is too high, you get resistance from the hormone receptor sites and it requires more of the hormone to create the same effect. Every cell in the body has receptors for both cortisol and thyroid hormones and nearly every cellular process requires optimal functioning of the thyroid.

It is common for women to have symptoms of an over- or under-active thyroid, particularly during perimenopause and menopause. If the situation is addressed at this point, further depletion of both thyroid and adrenal function can be prevented. If not, most women will be given estrogen replacement for their complaints, which further shuts down the thyroid. High estrogen levels interfere with thyroid hormones, particularly the utilization of T3, the most biologically active thyroid hormone.

More on the Thyroid Gland

In general, hypothyroidism or low thyroid hormone is a common condition in North America and affects between 20-25% of the female population and about 10% of males. In addition, approximately 30% of people over the age of 35 may have sub-clinical or mild hypothyroidism where the thyroid-stimulating hormone (TSH) from the pituitary gland is within the normal range but they have many symptoms of low thyroid.

Most doctors only test the TSH level and consider the thyroid function to be normal if the TSH falls between .4-4.2 IU/ml. However, naturopathic doctors and some medical doctors are using a new "norm" for the TSH lab value (between .4-3.0 IU/ml) and will treat for hypothyroidism if the person has accompanying symptoms. Remember the ideal TSH range is considered 1.0-2.0. It is also important to measure the level of the actual thyroid hormones T4 and T3 to get a more accurate picture of the function of the thyroid. TSH alone and the old lab values are inadequate and many hypothyroid patients suffer needlessly for years.

Some of the Common Symptoms of Hypothyroidism
▸ Cold hands and feet, cold intolerance, low body temperature
▸ Constipation
▸ Fatigue, weakness, lethargy
▸ Swelling of eyelids or face
▸ Depression and irritability
▸ Hair loss; dry, coarse hair or skin; cracking in the heels
▸ Hormonal imbalances (fibroids, ovarian or breast cysts, infertility, miscarriage, painful periods, endometriosis, menopausal symptoms, heavy periods or PMS)
▸ Impaired memory and poor concentration
▸ Slow metabolism – weight gain
▸ Goiter
▸ Heart palpitations
▸ Insomnia; racing thoughts
▸ Poor vision

An underactive thyroid may also result in elevated cholesterol levels and low progesterone-to-estrogen ratio, both of which are common in menopausal women.

Some Causes of Thyroid Problems
Hashimoto's thyroiditis is the most common hypothyroid condition. The autoimmune process attacks the thyroid and eventually the thyroid does not produce enough thyroid hormone. The treatment of hyperthyroidism using radioactive iodine and surgery is the second most common cause of hypothyroidism. Other causes include decreased use of iodized salt, increase in stress levels, anemia, estrogen replacement, birth control pills and other medications that block iodine uptake, and are associated with an increase in the number of people with hypothyroidism. In addition, for people living in the northern hemisphere, it is difficult to get adequate amounts of sunshine to produce vitamin D, a cofactor in thyroid hormone production. More and more studies and literature are coming out on the importance of vitamin D supplements for a myriad of conditions.

Maintaining optimal function of the adrenal glands and thyroid is a central part of a healthy transition through menopause.

Thyroid Health Tips

The thyroid gland requires the trace element iodine for the production of thyroxine (T4). Good sources of iodine include the sea vegetables (nori, hijiki, wakame, kombu and kelp), sea salt, saltwater fish and seafood. Some foods called goitrogens can interfere with proper iodine absorption, thus making it unavailable to the thyroid gland in the production thyroid hormones T4 and T3. Goitrogens are found in cruciferous vegetables (such as cabbage, turnips, broccoli, kale and mustard greens), soybeans, peanuts, pine nuts and millet. It is not essential to completely eliminate all goitrogens; just eat them in moderation.

Nutritional Supplementation for the Thyroid

▶ *Tyrosine* is an amino acid precursor to several neurotransmitters in the brain: dopamine, norepinephrine and epinephrine. These neurotransmitters are produced by the adrenal glands and are released in response to stress by the sympathetic nervous system. If tyrosine levels are drained, the adrenal glands cannot respond to stress adequately and there is less available to help make thyroid hormones.
Suggested use: 250-750 mg/day

▶ *Guggul (Commiphora mukul)* has been reported in studies to stimulate thyroid function.

▶ *Bladderwrack (Fucus vesiculosus)* is an algae that has been used medicinally in Europe and Asia for thousands of years. It is a rich source of iodine and has been used for weight loss and hypothyroidism.

▶ *ThyroSense*® is a natural combination of essential nutrients that support healthy hormone balance and the conversion of T4 to T3 (two hormones that are essential for regulating metabolism). ThyroSense also supports energy and healthy weight loss.
Suggested use: 2 capsules with breakfast

HRT – To Do or Not To Do??

Hormone replacement therapy (HRT) has been a popular course of treatment for many women with menopausal symptoms, but the decision to use HRT is a difficult one. HRT was originally developed to halt the symptoms of menopause but doctors also used it to prevent cardiovascular disease and to primarily prevent bone loss, but also in the treatment of depression, urinary incontinence, Alzheimer's disease and libido problems. No randomized, controlled clinical trials were ever conducted to verify if it could be used safely for these conditions. In July 2002, the results of the first randomized, controlled clinical trial – *The Women's Health Initiative Study* – concluded that the combination of estrogen and progestins posed a significant health risk to women and that the benefits of HRT are not worth the risk. Some of the dangerous side effects of HRT include the increased risk in breast cancer, cardiovascular disease, stroke and blood clots. Natural alternatives – including herbal products, nutrition and lifestyle – are quickly becoming the preferred choice over the controversial HRT. This awareness and education of HRT alternatives needs to be promoted in order for women to make educated decisions about their treatment options.

Diet and Lifestyle Changes

Nutrition and diet can greatly influence menopause and menopausal symptoms. One of the most important dietary recommendations for all menopausal women may be to increase foods that are high in phytoestrogens. Phytoestrogens are plant versions of the human hormone estrogen. They're considered to be weak estrogenic compounds with an average of about 2% of the strength of estrogens. They can be beneficial when estrogen levels are either too high or too low. When metabolized, they bind on the same cellular sites as do estrogens, altering estrogenic effects. The best food sources of phytoestrogens are non-genetically engineered soybeans, flax seeds, oats, rye, lentils, fennel, chick peas, alfalfa and sesame. Much research shows that women in Asia experience less menopausal symptoms because their diet contains a higher concentration of phytoestrogens, compared to women who adopt a North American diet.

Our North American diet is also typically deficient in essential fatty acids (EFAs), which are very important in many health conditions, ranging from inflammation and PMS to menopausal symptoms. Supplementing with essential fatty acids from flax or better yet from a good quality fish oil rich in omega-3s will also help with various menopausal symptoms.

Other Important Health Tips to Include:

- ▶ Eat a diet rich in cruciferous vegetables (broccoli, Brussels sprouts, cauliflower, cabbage and kale). Cruciferous vegetables contain Indole-3-carbinol and sulforaphane, important nutrients for maintaining balanced hormones in our liver while reducing our risk of breast cancer.
- ▶ Eliminate food sensitivities, as hot flashes can be reduced by 50% if sensitive foods are removed.
- ▶ Eliminate carbonated beverages as too much phosphorus competes with calcium absorption and the carbonation causes the body's pH to become acidic thus increasing bone resorption.

▸ Try to consume organic meats wherever possible (no hormones, byproducts or antibiotics). The estrogen in animal meats will bind tightly to estrogen receptors encouraging breast cancer.

▸ Eliminate caffeine, cigarettes, alcohol and sugar. These foods create an acidic environment in the body and thus calcium is leached out of the bone to balance the body's pH.

▸ Minimize exposure to exogenous estrogens: HRT, pesticides, herbicides, plastics and hormones used to fatten livestock and promote milk production (meats and dairy).

▸ Increase complex carbohydrates (fiber) which aids in the elimination of xenoestrogens.

▸ EXERCISE!!! Aerobic and weight bearing exercises improve heart function, decrease bone loss, give relief from hot flashes, reduce blood pressure, decrease cholesterol, and increase mood and energy.

After you have corrected your nutritional intake by your choice of food and lifestyle changes, choose supplements and herbs wisely. Strategies should include ways to balance fluctuating hormone levels, support the adrenal glands and prevent the risk for osteoporosis and heart disease.

The following are important nutrients and herbs for women during their menopausal years:

▸ *Stress B Formula (B-complex)* has a calming effect. It helps your body deal with stress and replenishes the adrenals. It supports a healthy nervous system and mood, promotes energy and helps counteract cravings for sweets.
Suggested use: 1 tablet/day

▸ *Vitamin C* with bioflavonoids helps diminish hot flashes and night sweats as well as support the adrenals, liver and immune function. Vitamin C also protects against cardiovascular disease and cancer.
Suggested use: minimum 1,000-4,000 mg/day or until bowel tolerance

▸ *Vitamin E* with selenium has a normalizing effect on estrogen levels. Vitamin E is good for hot flashes, breast tenderness, muscle cramps, vaginal dryness and will protect against heart disease, too.
Suggested use: 400-800 IU/day

▶ *Calcium/magnesium/vitamin D* supports bone health, muscle relaxation and cardiovascular health.
Suggested use for calcium/magnesium: see chapter on adrenal stress and bone metabolism
Suggested use for vitamin D: 2,000-4,000 IU/day

▶ *Black cohosh* is one of the more popular herbs used today to help ease symptoms of menopause such as PMS and hot flashes.
Suggested use: 160-320 mg of powdered extract/day

▶ *Chaste tree berry* is another herb widely used today to help balance hormones and minimize symptoms associated with hormone imbalances in women from premenstrual through menopausal ages.
Suggested use: 160-320 mg of powdered extract/day

▶ *Dong quai* (also known as angelica) helps relieve hot flashes, vaginal dryness and has been traditionally used to support uterine health.
Suggested use: 200-400 mg of powdered extract/day

▶ *Red clover blossom* will help detoxify the liver (essential for hormonal balance) and enhance the immune system as well.
Suggested use: 300-500 mg extract

▶ *MenoSense*® contains black cohosh, dong quai, chaste tree, hesperidin and gamma oryzanol. This formula supports and balances hormones, as well as reduces hot flashes and night sweats.
Suggested use: 2 capsules with breakfast

▶ Please refer to the sections on insomnia, depression and dementia/poor memory for treating any of these conditions that you may be experiencing during menopause.

THE MISSING LINK – SUPPORTING THE ADRENALS IN MENOPAUSE

As stress follows us for most of our life, once women hit menopause, another major stress becomes a reality. The hormonal fluctuations are a transitional period for women and require the proper support of the adrenal glands to ease menopausal symptoms. As mentioned before, the adrenal glands are key players in menopause and take over the production of sex hormones when the ovaries shut down.

AdrenaSense® provides herbal support for healthy adrenal glands to help women transition into menopause naturally and easily.

Please remember that each woman is an individual with individual hormonal fluctuations so what might work for one person might not work for another. It is always important to seek the guidance of a licensed health care practitioner when using the above herbs and supplements.

CHAPTER 6

Adrenal Stress and the Immune System

Stress has been implicated in causing a deficient immune system. Scientists know that psychological stress can affect the immune system, the body's defense against infection and disease including cancer. When we are stressed, our bodies go into a stress response, a fight-or-flight reaction, and – if prolonged – the body will shut down the non-essential bodily functions such as the immune system. During a stressful situation our immune system is not considered important for survival.

When we are exposed to stress over a period of time, be it emotional, physical, environmental or nutritional stress, our body sends out stress hormones. Stress can have negative effects on several immune factors such as interleukin-6 (IL-6), an inflammatory immune factor that causes inflammation, pain, swelling and an exacerbation in autoimmune diseases. IL-6 also causes calcium loss from the bones, which can lead to osteoporosis and osteoarthritis. Researchers have found that prolonged stress can also be associated with up to a 50% reduction of NK (natural killer) cells. NK activity plays a vital role against viral infection and fights cancer cells. Similarly nerve growth factor (NGF) is increased in people who are under stress and NGF inhibits the ability of disease-fighting cells to ward off infection. Prolonged stress with all of the chain reactions in the immune system can cause acute reactions such as cold or flu, inflammatory conditions or more chronic disease such as cancer. Stress hormones as well as psychological factors such as feeling helpless or suppressing negative emotions, can affect the growth and spread of cancerous tumors.

Conversely, there is evidence that a depressed HPA axis, resulting in too little corticosteroid, can lead to a hyperactive immune system and increased risk of developing autoimmune diseases – diseases in which the immune system attacks the body's own cells. Overactivation of the antibody-producing B cells may aggravate conditions like lupus, which result from an antibody attack on the body's own tissues.

STRESS TEST TO DETERMINE IMMUNE STATUS

- ☐ Unusual tiredness and/or dizziness 3
- ☐ Unexplained irregular heartbeat or shortness of breath 3
- ☐ Smoke, drink alcohol, caffeine or take prescription drugs 3
- ☐ Sugar or aspartame consumption 3
- ☐ Headaches and or muscle tension/joint pain 3
- ☐ Lack of sexual desire 3
- ☐ Nausea or irritable bowel/digestive problems 3
- ☐ Overexercising (more than 4x week) or no exercise 3
- ☐ No vitamin or mineral supplements 2
- ☐ Poor diet/fast foods 2
- ☐ Feelings of guilt 2
- ☐ Anxiety or depression 2
- ☐ Feeling overwhelmed a lot of the time or feeling trapped......... 2
- ☐ Being self-critical or lacking confidence 2
- ☐ Feelings of inadequacy or never being able to please 2
- ☐ Fear of getting a disease such as cancer 2
- ☐ Using antibacterial products/soaps................................. 1
- ☐ Not wanting to socialize, becoming more introverted 1
- ☐ Suppressed anger.. 1
- ☐ Inability to relax 1
- ☐ Fidgeting or restlessness 1
- ☐ Excessive appetite or loss of appetite 1
- ☐ Loneliness... 1
- ☐ Insomnia or poor quality sleep 1

Total Score: _____

How did you score? If you scored 12 or over, you are putting yourself at risk for immune system overload. Between 6 and 12 you are still coping with the stress in your life but you need to slow down. Between one and five you are in the peak range for stress management and if you keep this pace, you will reach the finish line healthy.

HEALTH TIPS FOR THE IMMUNE SYSTEM
Food that Harms, Food that Heals

Sugar is one food that should come with a warning label stronger than that found on cigarette packages. Sugar causes our natural killer (NK) cells to become inactive. As little as one teaspoon of sugar shuts off NK cells for up to six hours leaving us vulnerable to infectious disease or cell mutations. While sugar is toxic to the immune system fresh fruits and vegetables, nuts and seeds optimize it. Organic foods over pesticide laden foods should be chosen as much as possible and fresh wild fish, lean free-range chicken and turkey, along with a mild to moderate intake of red meat and purified water should make up the bulk of our diet.

Nutrients to Support Immune Function

▶ *Vitamin A* helps prevent colds and flus, repairs mucous membranes and enhances T-cell counts.
Suggested use: 1,500-3,000 IU/day

▶ *Vitamin C* helps to prevent allergies and has antiviral, antibacterial and anticancer properties.
Suggested use: 1,000-5,000 mg/day – in acute conditions. Take to bowel tolerance.

▶ *Vitamin E,* along with vitamin C and selenium, increases our resistance to infection and protects us against the damaging effects of stress. It also enhances T cell function and the release of the "good guy" immune factors.
Suggested use: 200-400 IU/day

▶ *Magnesium* is required for over 300 enzymatic reactions in the body and this alone makes it important to the immune system.
Suggested use: 100-200 mg/day (more with inflammatory conditions such as fibromyalgia)

▶ *Zinc* is truly the most important immune mineral and supports the thymus gland, the conductor of the immune system. Zinc also has antiviral and antibacterial properties.
Suggested use: 15-30 mg/day

▶ *Selenium* is required to fight off bacteria and viruses and ensure our T cells and NK cells work well. Selenium deficiency is considered to be a cause of cancer.
Suggested use: 200 mcg/day

▶ ***Coenzyme Q10*** has been found to halt tumor growth, have antibacterial and antiviral properties.
Suggested use: 30 mg/day

▶ ***Reduced glutathione*** is a regenerator of immune cells and a valuable detoxifying agent.
Suggested use: 45 mg/day

▶ ***Vitamin D*** hormone has been shown to increase the activity of natural killer (NK) cells and macrophages. It also has antimicrobial properties against viruses, bacteria and fungi.
Suggested use: 1,000-3,000 IU/day

▶ ***AdrenaSense*** supports the adrenal glands during periods of stress, thereby supporting the immune system.
Suggested use: 2 capsules midday with food

CHAPTER 7

Adrenal Stress and Breast Cancer

Breast cancer is the leading cause of death in women ages 35 to 54 and today, 1 in 8 women will get breast cancer and of those, 1 in 4 will die from the disease. Eighty percent of all cancers are thought to be related to environmental factors, while diet plays a role in at least 35% of all cancers. The risk factors outlined by the American Cancer Society include hereditary (genetics), starting menstruation early and going through menopause late (too many years of estrogen exposure) and a high fat diet. There are more common but less publicized risks for breast cancer: estrogen replacement therapy with prolonged use; oral contraceptives in young women with prolonged use; pre-menopausal mammography with early and repeated exposure; diets high in fat contamination with undisclosed carcinogens and estrogenic chemicals (xenoestrogens); exposure at home or the workplace to household cleaning chemicals as well as pollution from chemical plants and waste sites; excessive use of tobacco or alcohol; and lack of exercise.

A study of breast cancer patients assessed the individual's overall stress level and found that a high degree of stress predicted a decreased ability of NK cells to destroy cancer cells. As well, those with a high degree of stress showed a poorer response to interventions aimed at improving NK cell activity.

A study published in the *Journal of the National Cancer Institute* June 2000 found that women with advanced breast cancer who had high daytime levels of cortisol or those whose levels remained flat are significantly more likely to die sooner than patients with normal levels of the cortisol stress hormone. The researchers also found that the women with increased cortisol levels had fewer NK cells and the immune system was less able to fight the cancer cells.

Emotional and social stressors also influence the nervous and hormonal systems and have prognostic values due to the influence on the immune system. For years, it has been known that a positive outlook on life and people who adopt stress-coping skills have better immune function and lower cortisol levels. Recent studies confirm the positive benefits of guided imagery on psychological well-being and immune function in patients with breast cancer.

Also, women with breast cancer who have a "confidant" – someone they trust implicitly and can tell their deepest feelings to – deal with the diagnosis and treatment better and have an overall health improvement compared with women who do not feel safe to express their emotions. Expressing emotions helps to reduce stress that is bottled up inside.

BREAST CANCER RISK ASSESSMENT

Take the following breast health test and discover if you are at risk for breast cancer.

- ☐ Have not had children and are under 25 years of age 1
- ☐ Have not had children and are 25-35 years of age 1
- ☐ Have had no children and don't intend to 3
- ☐ Did not breastfeed 2
- ☐ Had an abortion of the first pregnancy 1
- ☐ Took birth control pills during teens or early 20s. A few months' use may increase risk by 30% and 10 years may double risk 3
- ☐ Taking or have taken HRT (Premarin, Provera, Prempro) 3
- ☐ Have had regular mammograms before menopause 2
- ☐ Don't exercise three times a week 2
- ☐ Have had depression taking tricyclic anti-depressants * 2
- ☐ Have breast implants (breast trauma) 1
- ☐ Had chest x-rays as teenager or during 20s 2
- ☐ Are exposed to EMFs due to excessive computer use or other .. 1
- ☐ Dye your hair with dark-colored dyes (source of xenoestrogens) 2
- ☐ Wear dry-cleaned clothing (source of xenoestrogens) 1
- ☐ Use bleached sanitary products eg. Tampons (xenoestrogens) .. 2
- ☐ Eat pesticide and herbicide-laden foods (xenoestrogen source) . 3
- ☐ Use nail polish remover containing toluene or phthalate 1
- ☐ Menstruation started before age of 12 2
- ☐ Late onset menopause after age of 54 2
- ☐ Eat a diet high in animal fat, dairy and meat (xenoestrogens source) 3

☐ Smoke, started early with excessive use 3

☐ Alcohol, started early with excessive use 3

☐ Don't eat cruciferous vegetables (e.g., broccoli, cauliflower, kale) 3

☐ Take cholesterol-lowering drugs which deplete CoQ10 3

☐ Use anti-hypertensives for lowering blood pressure
(decrease CoQ10) 3

☐ Using tranquilizers (studies show increase in breast tumors) 2

☐ Using ulcer medications which disrupt estrogen metabolism 2

☐ Are overweight or obese (fat stores estrogens) 3

☐ Use Flagyl for yeast infections (increases mammary tumors) 2

☐ Family history of breast cancer in mother, sister or daughter 1

Total Score: _____
0-18   Low risk
19-35   Moderate to high risk
36-65   High risk

We can choose alternatives to many of the risk factors mentioned above and we can make dietary and lifestyle changes that can help to reduce our risk of developing breast cancer.

The scope of breast cancer or cancer treatments is too vast to cover in this book but I can offer you tips on prevention.

Nutritional Tips
In general, try to include some of the basic immune system support remedies and dietary guidelines mentioned before. Also consider adding the following:

▶ *Indole-3 carbinol* (I3C) is a phytonutrient found in cruciferous vegetables. Research has shown that I3C helps break down estrogens to a non-toxic form. Suggested use: 150-300 mg/day

▶ *Calcium-D-glucarate* helps the liver remove excess estrogen from the body. Suggested use: 150-300 mg/day

▶ *Curcumin (turmeric)* is the chief ingredient found in curry and is one of the best herbs to support healthy inflammatory responses and help maintain cellular integrity. Suggested use: 2,000-3,000 mg/day

▶ *Green tea extract* contains polyphenols, catechins and flavonoids which are shown to support overall good health.
Suggested use: 1,000-2,000 mg/day

▶ *Lycopene* is a carotenoid found in tomatoes, pink grapefruit, papaya, guava and watermelon. It has been shown to support cellular health.
Suggested use: 5-10 mg/day

▶ *Sulforaphane* from broccoli sprout extract has been shown to support the body's natural detoxification processes, helping eliminate xenoestrogens.
Suggested use: 200-400 mg/day

All of the above ingredients are found in **EstroSense**®. For further support, you can add additional curcumin, green tea extract and sulforaphane to reach recommended suggested use.

▶ *Coenzyme Q10* has been shown to cause repression of breast tumors and prevent metastasis (spread of cancer) in some women.
Suggested use: 90-350 mg/day

▶ *AdrenaSense*® supports your system during times of stress and helps promote cellular integrity.
Suggested use: 2 capsules midday with food

What Else Can We Do?
It is not uncommon for women to put themselves last, taking care of everyone else's needs while sacrificing their own. What is more symbolic of the ability to nurture life than a woman's breast? Approximately 20-30% of the female patients in my practice have, or have had, breast cancer. Almost 100% of these women do not feel that their feminine nature has been or is being nurtured. It is up to each one of us to ensure that our own needs are met, to learn to communicate these needs to others and to make time in our lives to nurture ourselves.

CHAPTER 8

Adrenal Stress and Dementia and Alzheimer's Disease

According to the 2012 Alzheimer's Disease Facts and Figures, there are an estimated 5.2 million people in the U.S. living with Alzheimer's disease. One in 8 people over age 65 and nearly 50% over age 85 have Alzheimer's disease.

Women are more likely to develop Alzheimer's disease. A woman age 65 or older has a 1 in 6 chance of developing Alzheimer's disease in her lifetime, compared to 1 in 11 for a man.

The 35.6 million with dementia worldwide in 2010 is expected to double by 2030 to 65.7 million, and then nearly double again by 2050 to 115.4 million.

Alzheimer's disease is the leading form of dementia and represents 63% of all dementias. Vascular dementia is the second most common form and represents 20% of all dementias. Women represent 72% of the cases of Alzheimer's disease and 47% of vascular dementia cases.

EARLY SYMPTOMS OF DEMENTIA MAY INCLUDE:

▶ Memory loss affecting day-to-day function, such as forgetting phone numbers (even your own), appointments, a colleague's name and not remembering these things later.

▶ Difficulty performing familiar tasks such as preparing a meal or becoming so distracted that you forget to turn off the stove.

▶ Problems with language such as finding the right words, even simple words and making substitutions that do not make sense.

▶ Disorientation of time and place. It is normal to sometimes forget the day of the week but a person with dementia can become lost on their own street, not know how they got there or not know how to get home.

▶ Poor judgment such as wearing hot clothing on a warm day or not recognizing they have a condition that needs medical attention.

▶ Problems with abstract thinking such as balancing a checkbook or being able to pay bills or write a check for the right amount

▶ Misplacing things on a regular basis or putting things in inappropriate places such as the iron in the freezer

▶ Changes in mood, behavior or personality – people with dementia can start to exhibit mood swings, going from tears to anger for no apparent reason. A person can also become confused, suspicious or withdrawn, and apathetic or extremely fearful over nothing.

POSSIBLE CAUSES OF DEMENTIAS

▶ *Vascular dementia* is associated with decreased blood flow due to hardening of the arteries as well as dehydration, which can cause the blood to become sluggish or sticky, which restricts blood flow to the brain. Blood flow parameters are also decreased in patients with ischemic stroke.

▶ *Family history* – for some families, there is a definite connection between family history and dementias, though the connection to heredity is not fully understood.

▶ *The external environment* – contaminants such as heavy metals or pesticides and other chemicals in the water, soil or air are thought to be involved in dementias.

▶ *The internal environment* may be caused by nutritional deficiencies, a virus or problem with the immune system

▶ *Stress* – it has now been proven that stress has a direct effect on the development and progression of Alzheimer's disease through a part of the brain called the hippocampus. It is also hypothesized that a huge emotional shock (stress) can be a cause of this disease.

▶ *Amyloid protein* buildup is considered the hallmark of Alzheimer's disease but the drugs that remove these proteins so far have not succeeded in arresting the steady decline of thinking and memory.

Researchers believe that there is not a single cause of Alzheimer's but rather the cause includes a number of factors, different for each individual.

ALZHEIMER'S DISEASE/DEMENTIA AND THE STRESS CONNECTION

Have you ever noticed that your memory goes on vacation after you have been under a long period of stress? Researchers have found that high levels of cortisol, one of the main stress hormones produced during stress, has a negative effect on memory. Cortisol belongs to a family of stress hormones called glucocorticoids that, among other actions, can interfere with energy supply to brain cells involved in memory. The primary area of the brain that deals with stress is in the limbic system and because of its influence on emotions and memory is called the "emotional brain."

Deep within the limbic system lies the hippocampus. The fundamental functional role of the hippocampus in memory is widely recognized and has been the subject of current research in Alzheimer's disease as it represents one of the primary areas of degeneration in this disease.

Activation of the hypothalamic-pituitary-adrenal (HPA) axis is one of the hallmarks of Alzheimer's disease. Ongoing activation of the HPA axis enhances cortisol production, which is toxic to the hippocampal neurons. Elevated cortisol not only damages the hippocampus but it also reduces the inhibition of HPA, leading to a vicious cycle of increased cortisol production and further hippocampal damage. Thus, the catch-22 degenerative cascade begins and it can be very difficult to stop.

In a recent study at the University of California, it was found that when animals were injected for just seven days with dexamethasone, a glucocorticoid similar to the body's stress hormones, the levels of the different proteins in the brain increased by 60%. These proteins – such as beta-amyloid – aggregate and form plaques or tangles, another signature of Alzheimer's disease.

Stress hormones appear to rapidly exacerbate the formation of brain lesions and the progression of Alzheimer's disease. Management of both physical and psychological stress is crucial in the prevention and treatment of this devastating disease. So, stress and elevated stress hormones are erasing your memory, changing your emotions and erasing your brain cells… what can you do about it?

Nutritional Tips for Prevention and Treatment of Dementias and Dementia Risk

"Eating lots of nuts, fish and poultry while cutting down on red meat and butter could reduce the risk of Alzheimer's disease," reported the *New York Times*. The study, published in the journal *Archives of Neurology*, found those people with a diet that included more salads, good oils, nuts, fish, tomatoes, poultry, cruciferous vegetables and a lower intake of high-fat dairy products and red meat had a lower incidence of Alzheimer's disease.

The researchers were primarily interested in the overall consumption of several nutrients which previous research has suggested may affect Alzheimer's risk. These nutrients include saturated fatty acids (SFA), omega-3 polyun-saturated fatty acids (PUFAs), omega-6 PUFA, vitamin E, vitamin B12 and folate. Previous research had suggested that a greater intake of SFA could adversely affect cognitive function while increased intake of PUFAs, B12, folate and vitamin E is related to better cognitive function.

Yian Gu, a researcher at Columbia University in New York found that people who ate nutrients specifically selected for brain health had a 40% lower risk of developing Alzheimer's disease compared with others and that this diet is the easiest way to modify disease risk.

Aside:
I had read a Dutch study that said, "Backward locomotion appears to be a very powerful trigger to mobilize cognitive resource." Because my grandmother, my mother and my aunt all had varying degrees of dementia, I want to do all I can to prevent it from happening to me. So one day, I was walking up a hill backwards and a truck stopped and the driver asked what I was doing. I said, "I am trying to prevent Alzheimer's disease." The driver then said, "Too late!" Well, whether walking backwards will prevent Alzheimer's or not, it is a great way to use muscles you don't know you have and good for a few laughs, too.

Nutrients to Support Brain Health and Function

▶ *AdrenaSense®* in my opinion is the number one way to support brain health and memory because of the importance of managing stress.
Suggested use: 2 capsules midday with food

▶ *Alpha glycerylphosphorylcholine (GPC)* has been shown to be effective in reducing the loss of neuroconnecting fibers and brain cells. GPC is an extremely bioavailable source of choline, a building block of acetylcholine, which decreases with age. GPC has been linked with helping memory loss due to low acetylcholine levels. Studies have shown significant improvement in memory and overall function in patients with dementia.

▶ *Essential fatty acids* – Omega-3s are found in cold-water fish, such as salmon, sardines and mackerel. Omega-6s are found in seeds, nuts, some vegetable oils (including soybean, safflower, sunflower and corn oil), egg yolks and meats. Try to eat cold-water fish at least twice a week. At the same time, limit intake of omega-6s in processed and fried foods. Consider supplementing your diet with a good essential fatty acid supplement such as WomenSense® Rx Omega-3.
Suggested use: 2 softgels 1-3x/day

▶ *Turmeric* (curcumin) is a potent anti-inflammatory and anti-fibrin substance that helps clear toxic proteins involved in Alzheimer's disease.
Suggested use: 2,000-4,000 mg/day

▶ *Bacopa monnieri* is used in Ayurvedic medicine to enhance thinking and support memory function. It provides antioxidant protection for memory centers and reduces the effects of stress on the brain.
Suggested use: 200 mg 1-2x/day

▶ *Phosphatidylserine* is necessary for effective neurotransmission and is helpful in treating mental impairment such as Alzheimer's, dementia and depression.
Suggested use: 100 mg 2-3x/day

▶ *Vinpocetine (periwinkle)* increases blood circulation in the brain and reduces brain impairment and dementia after ischemic stroke. It also increases the concentration of neurotransmitters and is being used in the treatment of Alzheimer's disease.
Suggested use: 5-10 mg 3x/day

▶ *Ginkgo biloba* is a powerful antioxidant often associated with increased cerebral blood flow and enhanced memory.
Suggested use: 150-250 mg standardized extract/day

▶ *B12 and folic acid* – B12 promotes normal memory and verbal function and folic acid helps maintain normal homocysteine levels for healthy cognitive function.
Suggested use: B12 1,000–2,000 mcg/day (higher doses are used in Alzheimer's); Folic acid 1 mg/day

▶ *Vitamin E* has been shown to reduce the problems of memory loss and learning in the aging population by 36%. This result was published in the *Archives of Neurology*.
Suggested use: 400 IU/day

Exercise Prevents Mental Decline
New studies are providing even more evidence that regular aerobic exercise not only prevents problems with memory that come with aging but can actually help turn back the clock on brain aging. Researchers at the Mayo Clinic found that moderate exercise in mid-life was associated with a 39% reduced chance of developing cognitive impairment, and moderate exercise later in life

was associated with a 32% reduction in the odds of mental decline. Moderate exercise includes exercise such as brisk walking, aerobics, yoga, strength training and swimming. Try including one or more of these activities for 20 to 30 minutes 4 times a week into your regular routine. These studies published in the *Archives of Neurology* January 2010 contribute to a growing body of literature supporting the benefits of a physically active lifestyle in general but also on the brain.

Water
Keeping well hydrated is important for healthy brain function. Dehydration causes sticky or sluggish blood flow and less blood flow to the brain contributes to vascular dementia. Most people do not drink enough water so aim for at least eight glasses of filtered water daily.

Brain Games – Use It or Lose It
Brain fitness requires variety and curiosity. Most of us like familiarity but when anything you do becomes rote or second nature, then you need to make a change. Switch it up! Take a new route to work; go to a different grocery store; try a new type of exercise – try something new!

Brain fitness games are also a good way to challenge your brain: sudoku, crossword puzzles, Internet or electronic games, and card games like bridge can all exercise your brain. These games rely on logic, word skills, math and more. Try to find 15 to 20 minutes a day to exercise your brain.

Stress in Caregivers

The growing demographic within the baby boomers is referred to as the "sandwich generation." While elderly people are benefiting from rising life expectancies, their children – often parents themselves – are "sandwiched" in the middle, caring for two generations. Millions of Americans are caring for a loved one with a long-term health problem, which for many is a full time job on top of work and other family responsibilities.

A study was completed which focused on 119 men and women taking care of spouses with dementia. The health of the caregivers was compared with that of 106 people of similar ages not living under the stress of constant caregiving. The added responsibility as caregiver can have profound effects on mental, emotional and physical health as well as finances. Blood tests showed that a chemical called interleukin-6 (IL-6) was sharply increased in the blood of the stressed caregivers compared with blood of the other participants in the test. Previous studies have associated IL-6 with several diseases, including heart disease, arthritis, osteoporosis, type-2 diabetes and certain cancers.

The study also found the increase in IL-6 can linger in caregivers for as long as three years after a caregiver had ceased that role.

CHAPTER 9

Adrenal Stress and Depression, Anxiety and Insomnia

Depression is a very common condition and is becoming more and more prevalent in people of all ages. One in ten people in the U.S. has depression and it is the leading cause of disability in people ages 15 to 44. Depression affects approximately 14.8 million adults, or about 6.7% of the U.S. population age 18 and older in a given year. While major depressive disorder can develop at any age, the median age at onset is 32 and it is more prevalent in women than in men.

Anxiety disorders are the most common mental illness in the U.S., affecting 40 million adults age 18 and older (18% of the U.S. population).

An estimated 50-70 million U.S. adults have sleep disorders. Persons experiencing sleep insufficiency are also more likely to suffer from chronic diseases such as hypertension, diabetes, depression and obesity, as well as from cancer, increased mortality, and reduced quality of life and productivity.

The direct cause of depression is unknown but it is widely accepted that it is influenced by genetic, environmental, developmental and biochemical factors. The scope of this book does not allow an in-depth look at all the factors influencing depression and anxiety disorders. The focus of this book is the effects of stress on different conditions, so we will focus on the direct link of stress hormones and emotional disorders such as depression and anxiety.

THE "EMOTIONAL BRAIN" – LIMBIC SYSTEM

The primary area of the brain that deals with stress is the limbic system. Because of its enormous influence on emotions and memory, the limbic system is often called the "emotional brain."

Research studies have implicated disturbances in the serotonin (5-HT) system and the limbic hypothalamic-pituitary-adrenal (LHPA) axis as most consistently associated with mood-altering illness. The LHPA axis regulates arousal, sleep, mood, appetite and capacity to experience and enjoy pleasure. It has been strongly suggested that the interaction of these two biochemical systems play a significant role in depression.

The main brain chemicals (neurochemicals) and hormones that have been linked to the development of depression are namely norepinephrine, dopamine, serotonin, cortisol and thyroid hormones.

As previously mentioned, when the body is under stress, the adrenal glands increase the secretion of stress hormones called glucocorticoids. Cortisol is the main adrenal stress hormone that is regulated by the LHPA axis. The limbic system responds via the autonomic nervous system through a complex network of hormone secreting glands (endocrine glands).

In the short term, cortisol helps with survival. However, long-term elevation can have detrimental effects. Normally, cortisol levels peak in the morning and then decrease as the day progresses. In depressed people, the cortisol peaks earlier in the morning and does not level off or decrease in the afternoon or evening. There is little doubt that glucocorticoids have a profound effect on mood and behavior and that chronically elevated cortisol causes depression by affecting the serotonin receptor system. Researchers have found that once cortisol levels return to normal levels with treatment, depression disappears.

ANTIDEPRESSANT MEDICATIONS – A BRIEF OVERVIEW

Again, the scope of this book does not allow for an in-depth discussion about all the various medications available to treat depression. However, a brief explanation may shed some light on why some medications seem to work for some people while other medications do not.

Medications used to treat depression work in different ways. For example, the tricyclic antidepressants such as Imipramine work by regulating the LHPA axis and balancing the 5-HT system in the hippocampus and brain cortex. On the other hand, the selective serotonin reuptake inhibitor (SSRI) fluoxetine (Prozac) is unable to prevent the stress-induced elevation in cortisol and over-activity of LHPA axis. There is some evidence to show that persistently high levels of stress hormones (e.g., cortisol) – after the administration of antidepressant medication – is associated with relapse and poorer treatment outcomes in depressed patients.

Some clinical studies have found that the tricyclic antidepressants are more effective than the SSRIs in the treatment of melancholia, a severe form of depression characterized by complete loss of the capacity for pleasure. Patients with melancholia also tend to have high cortisol levels. For these patients and those with both depression and anxiety, it was found that Effexor, an antidepressant with both norepinephrine and 5-HT reuptake activity was reported to be more effective than Prozac.

It is very hard to know which antidepressant is going to be effective and it often requires a process of trial and error. One simple test that could be done to help determine the medication would be a salivary or blood cortisol level test.

This simple example may explain why some people are treatment-resistant to antidepressant medications.

ARE YOU DEPRESSED OR JUST "BLUE"?
Signs of Depression
It is normal to feel down or out of sorts some of the time and you may have wondered if you are depressed.

There are several kinds of depressive episodes and they can last months, or sometimes years, and they interfere with social and work functioning. According to the Diagnostic and Statistical Manual of Mental Disorders (DSM), to be considered depressed, you have at least five of the following symptoms:

- Depressed mood most of the day, nearly every day
- Markedly diminished interest or pleasure in all, or almost all activities
- Significant weight loss when not dieting or weight gain, or decrease or increase in appetite
- Insomnia or sleeping too much nearly every day
- Psychomotor agitation (unintentional motion caused from muscle tension)
- Fatigue or loss of energy almost daily
- Feeling of worthlessness or excessive or inappropriate guilt
- Diminished ability to think or concentrate or indecisiveness
- Recurrent thoughts of death, suicidal thoughts or attempt

However, whether you "fit" the depression diagnosis is not the most important thing. If you are feeling so down that you feel you need to do something about it, then that is what becomes the most important factor.

Only a qualified doctor or health practitioner can diagnose you with clinical depression.

ANXIETY AND PANIC ATTACKS
Along with glucocorticoids, the adrenal glands also secrete another class of hormones called catecholamines. Norepinephrine (NE) and epinephrine are the main catecholamines often associated with the fight-or-flight response to stress. NE can increase heart rate, blood pressure as well as create a sense of

overwhelming fear. (*See earlier section on physiology of adrenal glands*)

Low levels of NE are associated with loss of alertness or motivation, poor memory, ADHD and depression.

Elevated levels of NE – which can occur after prolonged stress – cause worry, anxiety, increased startle reflex, fears of crowds, jumpiness, impaired concentration, restless sleep or insomnia, muscle tension and irritability or edginess. Most anxiety symptoms are due to elevated NE levels. Severe and sudden increases in NE are associated with full blown "panic attacks."

The fight-or-flight response is a chemical reaction to a real or perceived life-threatening situation, where excess amounts of norepinephrine and epinephrine are produced which provide extra strength and increased energy needed to run or to fight. This reaction is needed for survival reactions like running from a bear in the woods. However, when these hormones become elevated during normal activity, they cause a panic or anxiety attack.

Glucocorticoids (GC) – particularly cortisol – also play important roles in fear and anxiety. The mechanisms by which GCs exert their effects on behavior are often indirect because, although corticosteroids do not regulate behavior, they induce chemical changes that determine certain behavioral outcomes. GCs can exert maladaptive rather than adaptive effects when their actions are chronically unbalanced due to chronic stress. The mental health of humans is likely to be seriously threatened after prolonged psychological or physical stress.

Anxiety/Panic Attacks Include the Following Symptoms:
- Palpitations, pounding or rapid heart rate
- Sweating and body temperature changes (chills/hot flashes)
- Trembling or shaking
- Shortness of breath
- Choking sensation
- Chest pain and discomfort
- Nausea or digestive distress
- Dizziness, lightheadedness or feeling faint
- Fear of losing control or going crazy
- Fear of dying
- Numbness or tingling

Nutrition Tips for Supporting Emotional Health and Well-Being
- ***Phosphatidylserine*** can offset the body's response to physical stress by decreasing the level of stress hormones. Researchers found that PS caused anxiety levels to decrease and helped alleviate stress-induced depression.
  Suggested use: 100-300mg/day

▸ *5-hydroxytryptophan (5-HTP)* – depression and anxiety have been linked to serotonin imbalances in the brain. 5-HTP may increase serotonin synthesis in these cases.
Suggested use: 100-200 mg 2-3x/day

▸ *St. John's wort (Hypericum perforatum)* extracts tested in the different trials were better than placebos and as effective as standard antidepressants for the treatment of mild to moderate depression and it had fewer side effects.
Suggested use: up to 300 mg/day (standardized to 0.3% hypericin)

▸ *Magnolia bark* contains biphenols which regulate the stress hormone cortisol and is helpful in reducing anxiety and anxiety related insomnia. Some supplements for the effective treatment of anxiety contain both magnolia and Phellodendron bark.
Suggested use: pill form 300-700 mg/day

▸ *Rhodiola rosea*, an adaptogen, increases resistance to a variety of biological and physical stressors and also offers anti-fatigue, anti-depressant and immune-enhancing effects. It improves the nervous system, helps insomnia and improves mental function.
Suggested use: 100 mg 2-3x/day

▸ *AdrenaSense®* contains many of the important adaptogenic herbs that help regulate stress hormones.
Suggested use: 2 capsules midday with food

▸ *Passionflower (Passiflora incarnata)* has been used as a folk remedy for anxiety and insomnia. Recent studies found passionflower to be comparable to benzodiazepine drugs (e.g., Ativan) in the treatment of anxiety and insomnia but had less drowsiness.
Suggested use: 200-400 mg/day

▸ *SAMe (S-adenosyl-L-methionine)* clinical trials in Europe and the U.S. have shown promising results in counteracting interferon-induced depression. Whereas antidepressants can cause liver damage, other studies on SAMe indicate it is liver protective.
Suggested use for depression: 400-1600 mg/day

INSOMNIA

Sleep and dreaming are essential to good health. Persons experiencing sleep insufficiency are also more likely to suffer from chronic diseases such as hypertension, diabetes, depression and obesity, as well as from cancer, increased mortality, and reduced quality of life and productivity. An estimated 50-70 million U.S. adults have sleep disorders.

Insomnia is a sleep disorder characterized by difficulty falling or staying asleep, or non-restorative sleep. Insomnia that occurs most nights and lasts a month or more is considered chronic insomnia.

Sleep is not a luxury, but rather an important component of health, no less so than air, water and food. Sleep is crucial for a vibrant, energetic and productive lifestyle and it is widely believed that seven to eight hours of sleep per night is necessary for optimal health.

Mark Mahowald, a professor at the University of Minnesota Medical School, states that one night of sleep deprivation is as impairing in simulated driving tests as a legally intoxicated blood-alcohol level. It has also been found that people who regularly do not get enough sleep have an increased risk for diabetes, hypertension, metabolic syndrome, obesity and premature aging.

Insomnia Related to Adrenal Dysfunction

Just like any other health condition, insomnia has many causes, ranging from psychological to biochemical to environmental factors. We will be focusing on the effects of stress on sleep problems.

To say that stress can affect proper sleep patterns seems obvious, but new research has found that sleep disturbances are directly related to increased sensitivity to arousal-producing stress hormones such as cortisol. Researchers compared patients with insomnia to those without sleep disturbances and they found that insomniacs with the highest degrees of sleep disturbance secreted the highest amount of cortisol, particularly in the evening and nighttime hours. Increased activation of the hypothalamic-pituitary-adrenal (HPA) axis – expressed as elevated plasma cortisol – is a main cause of primary insomnia.

Cortisol, the Anti-Sleep Hormone

The main stress hormone cortisol has a natural rhythm – normally peaking between 6:00 am and 8:00 am. Then between 8:00 am and 11:00 am, cortisol levels begin to drop and gradually decline throughout the day, reaching the lowest point about 2:00 am. The cyclical rise and fall of cortisol levels govern our level of wakefulness throughout the day and night. Cortisol is excitatory; it arouses us and wakes us up which is great in the morning. But, when as a result of prolonged stress cortisol levels get stuck at higher levels, that is bad news for a good night's sleep.

As a result of elevated nighttime cortisol, a person can feel extremely tired but unable to sleep. A common question asked by two-thirds of people with insomnia is, "If I am so tired, why can't I sleep?"

This common trend has been found in over two-thirds of the population who are experiencing chronic stress.

More and more studies are confirming that elevated evening cortisol due to stress is a main cause of chronic insomnia and sleep disturbances. Since nighttime exposure to increased HPA activity causes sleep problems, then regulation of the HPA axis and balance of the stress hormones is absolutely crucial for a good night's sleep and prevention of chronic disease related to sleep deprivation.

The Cortisol-Melatonin Relationship

In adults, the melatonin onset typically occurs during low cortisol secretion, which under normal circumstances would be at night. However, as mentioned previously, chronic stress causes an increase in cortisol in the evening, result-ing in decreased secretion of melatonin, one of the body's sleep hormones. Also, with aging, the production of melatonin declines and is shifted to later hours, while the production of cortisol increases and its peak occurs earlier in the night. Perhaps this is where the old wives tale that older people need less sleep comes from. It is not that the elderly need less sleep, it is simply that aging can cause dysregulation in the cortisol and melatonin secretions.

Insomnia Due to Shift Work

A person's work schedule also plays an important role in insomnia. Shift workers have insomnia three to four times the rate of non-shift workers. The hormones norepinephrine, epinephrine and dopamine are more elevated in people who have done shift work for more than five years. We covered earlier the consequences of elevated stress hormones and disease. Researchers found that the incidence of metabolic syndrome, cardiovascular disease, gastroin-testinal symptoms, menstrual irregularities and increased incidence of breast cancer is greater in long-term shift workers.

Blood Sugar Imbalances and Insomnia

Blood sugar imbalances are also a common – though less recognized – cause for insomnia. Adrenal compromised individuals commonly have blood sugar problems ranging from hypoglycemia (low blood sugar) to hyperglycemia (high blood sugar). Low blood sugar at night results in restless sleep, bizarre dreams and poor sleep quality for the entire night. One of the mechanisms the body will call on to liberate more glucose is to increase cortisol and adrenaline, which will convert stored fats and carbohydrates into sugars for immediate use. The increase in blood sugar sends more sugar to the brain, causing a restless, light sleep during the night. Coffee and alcohol exacerbate the problem while eating a small protein meal before bed can help regulate blood sugar levels.

Menopausal Insomnia
Another type of insomnia very commonly seen is sleep disturbances as a result of the menopausal transition. Some women wake up due to hot flashes at night, sometimes followed by episodes of chilling. For others, insomnia is independent of hot flashes. Once hormones are regulated, sleeping problems will improve for most women. (*see Menopause section*)

Health Tips for Insomnia Problems
General Tips: Start with these basic changes to restore restful sleep. If you need further support, see the remedies listed below.
- Cut out stimulants – avoid caffeinated beverages (coffee, tea, pop) past noon.
- Do not exercise in the evening as this can cause the cortisol levels to increase in people with adrenal fatigue.
- Do not eat a large meal late in the evening (after 7 pm). Try to avoid snacking after your dinner.
- Keep your fluid intake high during the day and less at night to avoid having to get up at night to urinate.
- Take time, one or two hours before bed, to write down all the "to do's" for the next day. Your mind will then settle more easily.
- Take a hot bath before bed (unless it aggravates hot flashes if you are a menopausal woman.) You can add essential oils such as lavender and chamomile.
- Take time for meditation, contemplation or prayer before you retire.

Support for Restful Sleep
- *Melatonin* helps to maintain the body's circadian rhythm, an internal 24-hour "clock" that plays a critical role in when we fall asleep and when we wake up. The body produces more melatonin when it is dark and decreases when it is light. Being exposed to bright lights too late in the evening can disrupt melatonin production.

▶ *Ginkgo biloba* has been found to inhibit stress-induced hormones via a mechanism involving adrenal benzodiazepine receptors. Further, ginkgo has been noted to prevent promotion of CRH (corticotropin-releasing hormone) seen in stress and blood sugar imbalances.

▶ *Phosphatidylserine* has been shown to reduce elevated cortisol levels.
Suggested use: 100 mg 2x/day

▶ *5-HTP* may prove to be better than melatonin. Several clinical studies have shown 5-HTP to produce good results in promoting and maintaining sleep in normal subjects as well as those experiencing insomnia. In many cases, insomnia has been associated with tryptophan deficiency in the tissues of the brain. Tryptophan is the precursor to 5-HTP which is then converted into serotonin and then into melatonin. Therefore, 5-HTP is a useful remedy for insomnia.

▶ *St. John's wort (Hypericum perforatum)* has been shown to have a positive effect on serotonin, dopamine and GABA receptors. Insomnia related to anxiety and depression may be effectively treated with this herb.
Suggested use: Start with 300 mg and you can take up to 900 mg if needed

▶ *Passionflower (Passiflora incarnata)* contains alkaloids that are muscle relaxing and an important flavonoid called chrysin which is also reported to bind benzodiazepine/GABA receptors in the central nervous system.
Suggested use: 200-400 mg solid extract one hour before bed or during the evening

▶ *Valerian (Valeriana officinalis)* contains a monoflavonoid called wognonin which is credited with the calmative effects of this classic sleep herb. Valerinic acid binds to GABA receptors and promotes relaxation and improved sleep.
Suggested use: 400-700 mg solid root extract one hour before bed. I suggest the capsules rather than the tincture as the latter's taste is enough to put most people off, unless you like the flavor of dirty socks.

▶ *Skullcap (Scutellaria lateriflora)* has wogonin and other flavones noted to bind to GABA receptors to promote sleep and relaxation. Note that benzodiazepines – a common class of sleep drugs – work by binding to GABA receptors as well.
Suggested use: 3-6 grams/day

▶ *Hops (Humulus lupulus)* is a phytoestrogenic herb and is very helpful for insomnia related to menopause. In the past, "hops pillow" was popular for promoting sleep. You can make a tea from hops and have one or two cups before bed. It doesn't taste great but helps with sleep.
Suggested use: 1 tsp hops to 2 cups boiled water, steep for 15 minutes

▶ *AdrenaSense®:* The adaptogenic herbs in **AdrenaSense®** will help to regulate the stress hormones and, in time, sleep will improve. For immediate help, try the other remedies listed to help you fall asleep. Once your adrenal glands are regulated, you should no longer need additional help with sleep.
Suggested use: 2 capsules midday with food. Do not take with dinner.

CHAPTER 10

Adrenal Stress and Allergies

Itchy eyes, runny nose, upset stomach, joint pain and skin rashes…most of us have experienced these symptoms or have a friend or family member who suffers from them.

Allergies are becoming more and more rampant. The number of North Americans suffering from asthma, hay fever, eczema and food allergies has reached unprecedented levels. For example, the number of people in the U.S. who have either allergy or asthma symptoms are one in five. Allergies also come with a hefty yearly price tag. The percentage of the U.S. population that tests positive to one or more allergens is 55% with an estimated cost to the health care system and businesses of 7.9 billion annually. Food and environmental allergies have been implicated in a wide range of medical conditions affecting virtually every part of the body and can manifest as either the symptoms above (skin rashes, stomach problems and itchy eyes), as more serious ones such as disorders of the central nervous system (depression, anxiety and chronic fatigue) or autoimmune diseases such as rheumatoid arthritis and lupus.

Common Indications of Allergies
- Depression, anxiety, insomnia
- Respiratory – asthma, chronic bronchitis
- Skin conditions – eczema, psoriasis, rosacea, dermatitis, acne
- Attention deficit disorder with hyperactivity
- Autism
- Inflammatory diseases – joint pain, low back pain, arthritis, chronic fatigue syndrome, fibromyalgia, lupus

▶ Gastrointestinal diseases – ulcerative colitis, Crohn's disease, irritable bowel syndrome, candida, ulcers, gastric reflux disease, diarrhea, constipation, celiac, canker sores
▶ Migraine headaches
▶ Multiple sclerosis
▶ Immune dysfunction – ear infections, chronic infections such as the flu, respiratory/sinus, chronic swollen glands and fluid retention
▶ Dark circles and puffiness under the eyes ("allergic shiners")
▶ Genitourinary – bed-wetting, chronic bladder infections
▶ Edema, fatigue, hypoglycemia, itchy nose or throat, sinusitis

THE ROLE OF THE IMMUNE SYSTEM AND ALLERGIES

Allergies are a disorder of the immune system that is caused by an improper immune response.

There are two types of immunity the body develops to protect itself: innate immunity and acquired immunity.

▶ *Innate Immunity:* Consists of immune cells and mechanisms that defend and protect against infections and dangerous pathogens that might damage the human body.
▶ *Acquired Immunity:* Consists of the body's adaptive ability to develop a memory for potential invading pathogens such as bacteria, viruses and other toxins so when encountered, the immune system will recognize and mount a stronger immune response at each exposure of that specific pathogen.

Acquired immunity is involved in allergies and allergic reactions. Antigens are substances (such as food, bacteria or molds/dust) that initiate an immune response. Since food is something that we consume on a day to day basis, it is easy to appreciate why food represents one of the largest challenges that the immune system must deal with.

Allergies are almost always linked to the presence of an excessive amount of allergic antibodies.

Certain food allergens or inhaled particles (such as dust or tree pollen), when exposed to frequently, will trigger a defense mechanism whereby the immune system will release antibodies thus causing a wide variety of symptoms as mentioned above. Two commonly produced antibodies are IgG and IgE. IgG reactions occur over several hours or days whereas IgE reactions occur within minutes or hours of exposure. Seventy-five percent of the antibodies we produce are IgGs. The digestive system is also an important component when dealing with allergies because a large portion (70%) of your immune system resides in your gut! This is called the GALT (gut associated lymph tissue). When certain foods react with the GALT repetitively, inflammation results and over time will cause the intestines to become "leaky." As poorly digested foods and allergens are able to cross the "leaky" membrane and move into the bloodstream, IgE and IgG antibodies are produced, causing havoc on the immune system and resulting in a wide spectrum of allergy symptoms. IgA is another antibody that has a critical role in protecting the integrity of the gastrointestinal layer. It is mostly found in mucosal layers such as the nose, respiratory passages, digestive tract, ears, eyes and vagina. IgA antibodies protect the mucosal layers from foreign substances and infections.

Allergy Testing

Conventionally accepted medical approaches for allergy assessment may include skin scratch tests in which small punctures are made on the skin with needles containing tiny amounts of allergens. This type of testing is limited because it only tests for IgE (immediate) reactions in the body. A blood test called ELISA (enzyme-linked immunosorbent assay) is used to test both IgE and IgG reaction, therefore providing a detailed and comprehensive analysis to accurately determine both immediate and delayed food and environmental allergies.

Causes of Food Allergies

- ▶ Excessive consumption of certain food allergens (including dairy, gluten, egg, corn, soy)
- ▶ Exposure to a high level of preservatives, stabilizers, artificial colorings and flavors, pesticides, medications (antibiotics and corticosteroids) and hormones added to our foods
- ▶ Chemical pollution in the air, water and food
- ▶ Early weaning off and early introduction to certain foods as an infant
- ▶ GMO foods
- ▶ Impaired digestion – deficiencies in enzymes, good bacteria (acidophilus and bifidobacteria) or stomach acid can lead to protein maldigestion and eventual damage to the intestinal lining
- ▶ Genetic predisposition – a study was done and results showed that if both parents were allergic, there was a 67% chance that their children would be allergic as well
- ▶ STRESS!

ADRENAL STRESS AND ALLERGIES

During adrenal stress, cortisol plays an important role in regulating the immune system and the immune response. In fact, a conventional pharmaceutical approach to allergies and asthma is hydrocortisone, which is an artificial form of cortisol to help decrease inflammation and a heightened immune response. There is also overwhelming support that stress has a detrimental effect on the natural killer cells of the immune system. Natural killer cells are produced by lymphocytes (white blood cells) and help monitor and protect the body from viruses and cancer cells (see chapter on cancer and stress). Therefore continual stress does have a negative impact on the immune system's ability to function optimally and protect from potential pathogens and respond efficiently to antigens such as certain foods and environmental allergens.

Increased levels of cortisol can also impair the function of the immune system and the antibody IgA, a vitally important antibody that protects the cells of the intestine. With insufficient IgA antibodies, the gastrointestinal tract is vulnerable to foreign particles which can lead to immune reactions and thus food allergies/intolerances.

The adrenal glands help control blood sugar levels and regulate hydrochloric acid (HCl) secretion and motility of the gastrointestinal tract. During adrenal stress, increased cortisol can result in a decreased production of HCl and thus poor digestion and motility in the digestive tract. This can result in bloating, gas, constipation, heartburn and poor digestion of food. Adrenal stress can also have a significant influence on the balance of intestinal flora. Acidophilus and bifidobacteria are protective bacteria that reside in the small and large intestine and protect us from overgrowth of yeast, *E. coli* and other harmful bacteria.

Studies have shown that stress can substantially decrease levels of these protective bacteria in the gut.

Lifestyle and Diet Modifications for Allergies

▶ As mentioned above, because the digestive system plays such a key role in immune health, determining underlying food allergies and avoiding those foods is highly beneficial. Eliminate the most common allergens: dairy, gluten, egg, soy, peanuts and corn.

▶ Eliminate refined/junk foods as these foods put even more stress on an already stressed out immune system. Eating sugar decreases your white blood cell count for six hours after consumption.

▶ Eat more fresh fruits and vegetables (organic when possible), hormone-free animal products and whole grains such as brown rice, quinoa, millet and gluten-free oats.

▶ Ensure adequate sleep. Get at least 8 hours of sleep per night to allow your body time to regenerate so that your immune system may function optimally.

▶ Drink plenty of water. Dehydration is one of the most common causes of fatigue, headaches and constipation. Keeping your bowels moving regularly (meaning at least once per day) will help to reduce the toxic load on your body and protect your body's immune system. Add one or two tablespoons of ground flaxseed to your morning smoothie or porridge if you find you are not going as frequently as you should be.

▶ Include the following immune-boosting foods in your diet: garlic, ginger, onions, thyme, oregano, blueberries, broccoli, spinach, mushrooms (shiitake, reishi, etc.), and red and yellow fruits and vegetables like peppers, sweet potatoes and citrus fruits. Be sure to consume these foods in their whole form, meaning eat the orange, not orange juice.

Nutritional Supplementation for Allergies

▶ Supplement with the bioflavonoid quercetin, which has been shown to be effective in individuals suffering from allergies. Quercetin inhibits the release of histamines and other inflammatory compounds from mast cells, thus reducing the allergic/inflammatory response.
Suggested use: 500 mg 3x/day

▶ Take vitamin C, key in any allergy treatment program, since it has so many beneficial functions. Vitamin C not only acts as an antioxidant helping to reduce allergic reactions but it also has mast-cell-stabilizing properties that reduce histamine release.
Suggested use: at least 1,000 mg/day of buffered vitamin C or until bowel tolerance

▶ Support the intestines by re-establishing the "good bacteria" (acidophilus and bifidus) to ensure proper digestion of foods and optimal immune function. Digestive enzymes can also be beneficial in assisting with the proper digestion of protein, fat and carbohydrates, easing the digestion process through the gastrointestinal system.

▶ Essential fatty acids (omega-3 especially from fish and flax) will help decrease inflammatory and allergic reactions in the body.
Suggested use: minimum of 800 mg of EPA and 400 mg of DHA/day

▶ Supporting your adrenals can help promote healthy inflammatory responses.
Suggested use: **AdrenaSense**° 2 capsules midday with food

▶ The liver is an important organ to support when dealing with allergies as it is one of the main organs of detoxification. Use herbs such as dandelion and milk thistle to help properly eliminate toxins through the liver.

CHAPTER 11

Adrenal Stress and Bone Metabolism

BONE BUILDING BASICS

Bone is living tissue that is constantly being broken down and rebuilt. Bone metabolism involves the removal of old bone from the skeletal system (bone resorption) and the addition of new bone (ossification). This process controls the healing and remodeling of bone during growth and following injuries such as fractures and micro-damage, which can occur during normal activity. In the first year of life, almost 100% of bone is replaced. In adults, remodeling proceeds at a rate of about 10% per year. The cells responsible for creating new bone are called osteoblasts, while osteoclasts are the cells that break bone down. The structure of bone requires a close relationship and depends on the cooperation between these two cells. Adequate levels of calcium and other minerals, as well as complex signaling pathways, help achieve proper rates of growth. These signaling pathways include the action of several hormones, including the parathyroid hormone (PTH), vitamin D, growth hormone, steroids and calcitonin.

Osteoporosis is a bone disease that can result from an imbalance in bone metabolism. It occurs when bone is broken down faster than it can be rebuilt and over time, a gradual decrease in bone mass causes the bones to become porous, brittle and fragile, increasing the risk of fracture.

OSTEOPOROSIS

Osteoporosis is a degenerative disease involving the slow degradation of bone mass and integrity. This leads to increased bone fragility and risk of fracture, particularly of the hip, spine and wrist. It is often referred to as a "silent disease" because it develops slowly over many decades. In fact, many people don't even discover they have osteoporosis until they break a bone or crack a rib.

Osteoporosis is a global public health problem currently affecting more than 200 million people worldwide. In the U.S. alone, 10 million people have osteoporosis, and 18 million more are at risk of developing the disease.

Eighty percent of people who suffer osteoporosis are women. However commonly seen in women, the burden of osteoporosis in men remains underdiagnosed and underreported.

Let's look at the progression of bone growth throughout our lifetime. Bones will steadily grow in length and density until the later teens. After this time, bones will continue to increase in density but at a slower rate. Then, when you hit your 20s, bones achieve what's called their peak mass. This means that they stop building density and natural bone loss begins. Before menopause, women lose bone at a rate comparable to men (at a rate of 1% per year). But with the loss of estrogen at menopause, women will lose bone two to six times faster. The rate of bone loss returns to 1% per year 10 years after menopause.

Risk Factors

▶ Family history of osteoporosis
▶ Gastric or small-bowel resection (low absorption and assimilation of calcium)
▶ Sedentary lifestyle
▶ Heavy alcohol and tobacco use
▶ Hyperparathyroidism
▶ Hyperthyroidism
▶ Menopause
▶ Low calcium intake from diet
▶ Eating disorders
▶ Long-term use corticosteroid therapy, aromatase inhibitors to treat breast cancer, the antidepressant medications called selective serotonin reuptake inhibitors (SSRIs), the cancer treatment drug Methotrexate, some anti-seizure medications, the acid-blocking drugs called proton pump inhibitors and aluminum-containing antacids are all associated with an increased risk of osteoporosis
▶ Nulliparity (never having been pregnant)
▶ Short stature and small bones
▶ White or Asian race

Diagnosis

Osteoporosis is best diagnosed using dual energy x-ray absorptiometry (DEXA). DEXA is considered the "gold standard" because it exposes a person to considerably less radiation than other x-ray procedures. In the DEXA scan, measurements of both the hip and lumbar spine are taken.

Stress and Bone Metabolism

During periods of stress, the hormone cortisol is secreted from the adrenal glands. High levels of cortisol inhibit the cells that form bone (osteoblasts). Thus, over-production of cortisol results in the loss of bone density. For example, the use of corticosteroids (such as prednisone), which mimic the action of cortisol, will have the same effect on bone health. These drugs also decrease the amount of calcium that is absorbed from food and increase the amount of calcium lost in the urine. An increased production of cortisol is also very acidic and corrosive to our bones, forcing the body to leach vital bone building minerals from the bone to buffer the acidity in the blood and thus excreting those minerals in the urine.

Lifestyle and Diet Modifications for Osteoporosis

▶ Reduce the consumption of caffeine, alcohol and sugar. These foods create an acidic environment in the body and thus calcium and other minerals are leached out of the bones to buffer the body's pH to make it more alkaline.

▶ Eliminate all soft drinks; they contain phosphorus, which leaches calcium out of the bones, too.

▶ Minimize animal protein, such as red meat, as it contains high saturated fats which creates acidity in the body and can lead to calcium loss.

▶ Reduce salt. It increases calcium loss through the urine.

▶ Eat calcium-rich foods including green, leafy vegetables such as broccoli, collard greens, turnip greens, kale, dulse, dandelion greens, watercress, parsley, kelp, pinto, aduki, soybeans, tofu, almonds, hazelnuts, sunflower and sesame seeds.

▶ Reduce "bad fats" which promote bone loss (saturated fats, deep fried)

▶ Increase "good fats" which enhance bone density (omega-3s, fish and flax oils)

▶ Develop an adequate exercise program that includes weight-bearing as well as cardiovascular activities.

▶ Avoid antacids – they lower the acid in your stomach and inhibit the absorption of calcium.

Nutritional Supplementation for Supporting Healthy Bones

▶ *Calcium* helps strengthen bones during the building process and is fundamental for maintaining bone mass. At age 50, the requirement for calcium intake increases from 1,000 mg to 1,500 mg daily. There is a great deal of confusion and controversy about which form of calcium is best. The most absorbable forms of calcium are bound to citrate, fumarate and malate. Calcium carbonate seems to be the least absorbable form.

▸ *Vitamin D* is well known for its role in building strong bones and teeth; however a study published in *The American Journal of Clinical Nutrition* found that taking vitamin D supplements and calcium substantially reduces all cancer risk in post-menopausal women.
Suggested use: 1,000-4,000 IU/day

▸ *Magnesium* – When it comes to strong bones, magnesium supplementation may turn out to be as important as calcium.
Suggested use: 250-500 mg/day of magnesium citrate

▸ *Vitamin C* is an important antioxidant that helps support our immune system and plays an important role in collagen production, which in turn contributes to bone formation.
Suggested use: 1,000 mg of vitamin C/day for optimal bone health

▸ *Zinc* is an important mineral responsible for producing both osteoblasts and osteoclasts and has healing qualities during bone damage.
Suggested use: 15-30 mg/day

▸ *Strontium* is a trace mineral that is starting to gain more recognition for bone building. It supports the function of new bone growth while reducing the activity of bone breakdown. It is important not to take strontium together with your calcium supplement as both compete for absorption in the intestines. The best protocol is to take strontium 3 hours after your last meal (before bed) or 1 hour before breakfast.

▸ *Vitamin K2* can be used in conjunction with **BioSil®** to support strong, healthy bones.
Suggested use: 1 capsule/day

▸ Other important nutrients for bone health include boron, manganese, copper, potassium, essential fatty acids, ipriflavone and silica.

▸ *OsteoSense® Plus* will help promote bone formation, increase deposit of calcium into bone and promote healthy absorption of calcium. The ingredients include calcium, magnesium, zinc, copper, vitamin D, vitamin C and ipriflavone.
Suggested use: 1-2 tablets 2x/day

▶ *AdrenaSense®* is one of the foundations for healthy bones. **AdrenaSense** helps support the body during times of stress, especially during hormone fluctuations in menopause.
Suggested use: 2 capsules midday with food

▶ *BioSil®* is made of ch-OSA® (choline-stabilized orthosilicic acid), an important element for healthy bone density, bone mass, nails, joint cartilage, hair and skin.
Suggested use: 1 capsule daily or 6 drops daily

Osteoporosis is a preventable illness if appropriate dietary and lifestyle measures are followed. Women of all ages from very young to very old should make building healthy and strong bones a lifelong priority. This involves avoiding dietary and lifestyle practices that leach calcium from the bones, and choosing dietary factors that promote bone health.

CHAPTER 12

Adrenal Stress and Inflammation

Inflammation is a normal process of the human body. It is the first response of the immune system to infection, injury or irritation from a foreign substance. Perhaps the most common type of inflammation is acute, the kind you experience when you burn your hand while cooking, sprain your ankle while playing a sport or overuse your muscles while lifting heavy items. The body usually responds with redness, pain, swelling and warmth in the area.

Inflammation may also be associated with flu-like symptoms such as fever, chills, fatigue and aching in response to infection from a virus or bacteria such as the common cold or flu. When the immune system is performing normally, inflammation helps initiate the healing process. The inflammatory process is mediated by the release of certain inflammatory mediators including histamine, prostaglandins, cytokines such as C-reactive protein and interleukin-6 (IL-6), causing redness, swelling, warmth and pain. The purpose of the inflammatory response is to remove debris, attack foreign invaders, remove cellular waste and encourage the healing process.

Unfortunately, in chronic inflammation as seen in fibromyalgia or osteoarthritis, persisting inflammation leads to oxidative stress because of the over production of reactive oxygen and nitrogen species as well as the depletion of antioxidant molecules. Some reactive species such as free radicals can cause extensive cellular damage and in more severe cases even cause cell death. Some chronic inflammatory diseases include osteoarthritis/rheumatoid arthritis, heart disease, digestive disorders (Crohn's and ulcerative colitis) chronic fatigue syndrome, fibromyalgia and even cancer.

In some cases, the body's immune system can overreact or react inappropriately. In autoimmune diseases for instance, the body's normally protective immune system causes damage to its own tissues.

Lifestyle factors such as stress, poor eating habits and lack of sleep will all contribute to inflammation. While there are often obvious signs of acute inflammation, such as redness and swelling, chronic inflammation, which can occur over a long period of time from poor lifestyle factors, can be more subtle. Inflammation of this nature can affect many body tissues including blood vessels, organs and nerves with few or no obvious signs and symptoms until a serious health problem develops.

OSTEOARTHRITIS

About 50 million North Americans (approximately 1 in 7) have some form of arthritis. In another 20 years, as baby boomers grow older and people live longer, close to 70 million people in the United States and Canada will have arthritis.

The most common form of arthritis is osteoarthritis, also known as degenerative joint disease. Osteoarthritis occurs when the cartilage that cushions the ends of the bones in your joints deteriorates over time. This results in irritation in the joint and eventually if the cartilage wears down completely, you may be left with bone rubbing on bone thus increasing inflammation and pain.

While osteoarthritis can affect any joint in the body, the most commonly affected joints are:

- Hands
- Hips
- Knees
- Spine

Risk Factors

- Genetic predisposition
- Older age
- Fractures and mechanical damage
- Obesity
- Hormonal and sex factors
- Inflammatory joint disease such as rheumatoid arthritis (RA), gout, septic arthritis, etc.

ADRENAL STRESS AND THE INFLAMMATORY RESPONSE

During periods of stress, the hormone cortisol is released as a coping mechanism. Cortisol has potent anti-inflammatory properties which is particularly evident when it is administered pharmacologically as drugs (cortisone or prednisone) to treat inflammatory conditions like arthritis and as adjunctive therapy for conditions such as autoimmune diseases.

Cortisol blocks not only the initial inflammatory response but also the latter stages such as cellular proliferation of chronic inflammation. In small quantities, cortisol is very useful and essential in tissue repair, and controlling inflammation and excess immune cell production. But in chronic stress, elevated cortisol levels slow down the production of anti-inflammatory messengers thus resulting in inflammation and immune suppression. Eventually, when cortisol levels are depleted due to chronic stress, adrenal fatigue will allow the immune system cells to circulate in excess. This leads to the immune system attacking itself, resulting in autoimmune diseases such as RA and lupus.

FIBROMYALGIA

Fibromyalgia (FM) is a chronic and complex disorder that is often misunderstood – even sometimes unrecognized – that causes widespread musculoskeletal pain and tenderness that seems to move around the body. FM affects 5% of the population with approximately 90% of those diagnosed being women between the ages of 20-50 years of age. However, men, adolescents and children can also be diagnosed with this syndrome. There is a remarkable overlap between fibromyalgia and chronic fatigue syndrome which we will talk about in more detail later. Approximately 70% of patients diagnosed with fibromyalgia have the same diagnostic criteria for chronic fatigue syndrome (CFS).

Unfortunately, it often takes a long time before a person is correctly diagnosed with FM. The patient usually undergoes a series of medical investigations and tests over many years before being diagnosed. This delay is often due to the general physician's over-investigation of the multiple individual symptoms that the patient presents with rather than looking at the big picture of FM.

There are multiple theories regarding the development and causes of FM. It is very likely that there are certain types of genes that can predispose people to developing fibromyalgia and other co-existing conditions. However, genetics alone do not cause FM; often there is some trigger such as arthritis, spinal disorders, illnesses/infections, physical or emotional stressors and low serotonin levels that can play a role as well.

Diagnosis

The American College of Rheumatology has established two major criteria for the diagnosis of FM:

▶ Generalized aches or stiffness in all four quadrants of their body for a minimum of three months.
▶ At least 11 positive tender points out of a total possible of 18.

While there is no lab test to confirm a diagnosis of fibromyalgia, blood tests may be performed to rule out other conditions with similar symptoms.

Blood tests may include complete blood count, erythrocyte sedimentation rate and thyroid function tests.

Minor criteria may include:
▸ Generalized fatigue
▸ Sleep disturbances
▸ Joint swelling
▸ Chronic headaches
▸ Cognitive and memory problems
▸ Symptoms of depression and anxiety
▸ Irritable bowel syndrome
▸ Numbing and tingling sensations
▸ Irritable bladder

The symptoms of fibromyalgia can vary in strength, from person to person and will wax and wane over time. Stress is often a big culprit and often worsens these symptoms. As mentioned above, there is a lot of overlap in diagnostic criteria between CFS and FM; the biggest difference however to be noted is the requirement of musculoskeletal pain in FM and fatigue in CFS.

Fibromyalgia, Adrenal Stress and Serotonin

There are many contributing factors connected to FM but one interesting theory is a low level of serotonin and tryptophan which can cause the sensation of pain to be greatly exaggerated. Some studies have shown symptomatic improvement (stiffness, anxiety, fatigue and pain) with the use of tricyclic and SSRI antidepressants (increasing the levels of serotonin in the bloodstream).

5-hydroxytryptophan (5-HTP) is the immediate amino acid produced in the body from the essential amino acid L-tryptophan (LT) in the biosynthesis of serotonin. In the central nervous system, serotonin levels have been implicated in the regulation of depression, sleep, anxiety, appetite, pain and sexual behavior. Therapeutic administration of 5-HTP has been shown to be very useful in the treatment of fibromyalgia, depression, anxiety, insomnia and chronic headaches.

Adrenal stress can lead to decreased levels of LT and 5-HTP in the bloodstream from increased cortisol levels as well as a deficiency of vitamin B6, which is an important cofactor in the production of serotonin from 5-HTP. Eventually, chronic stress will lead to adrenal fatigue whereby cortisol levels decrease and chronic inflammation and pain is inevitable.

Nutritional Supplementation for Fibromyalgia
▶ *5–HTP* can be effective for individuals with fibromyalgia. By enhancing serotonin levels, symptoms of anxiety, insomnia, depression and pain can be greatly diminished.

CHRONIC FATIGUE SYNDROME

Chronic fatigue syndrome (CFS) is a complicated disorder characterized by persistent fatigue that may worsen with physical or mental activity, but does not improve with rest. It is estimated that as many as 800,000 adults in the U.S. may have CFS. Fewer than 20% of these individuals will have been diagnosed with CFS and received medical attention for their fatiguing illness.

The overall prevalence of CFS was 235 per 100,000 persons and it is 4 times more common among women than men. It is also most common among white women 50 to 59 years of age. On average, the illness lasts about 7 years. CFS is a multisystem disease affecting the nervous, immune and endocrine systems.

Other symptoms may include:
▶ Widespread muscle and joint pain
▶ Low grade fever
▶ Cognitive difficulties
▶ Recurrent headaches
▶ Sleep disturbances
▶ Depression
▶ Tender lymph nodes
▶ Recurrent sore throat
▶ Digestive problems
▶ Poor immune response

As mentioned before, CFS symptoms can overlap with those of fibromyalgia (FM).

Although there are many theories about what causes this condition, several possible causes have been proposed, including:
▶ Depression
▶ Iron deficiency anemia or other nutritional deficiencies
▶ Some prescription drugs (antihypertensives, anti-inflammatories, birth control pill, antihistamines and corticosteroids)
▶ Hypoglycemia (low blood sugar)
▶ History of food allergies
▶ Virus infection, such as Epstein-Barr virus or human herpes virus 6

▶ Pre-existing physical condition (diabetes, heart disease, chronic pain, inflammation, etc.)
▶ Stress/low adrenal function
▶ Impaired liver function
▶ Hypothyroidism
▶ Sleep disturbances

Adrenal Stress and CFS

Stress is an important factor to consider when dealing with CFS. In end stage adrenal fatigue, low levels of cortisol create symptoms of extreme and debilitating fatigue. Adrenal stress can also be an underlying factor in a patient with depression (as discussed in the depression chapter), low immune function, hypothyroidism, hypoglycemia, food allergies as well as many other causes of chronic fatigue.

Nutritional Supplementation for Healthy Nervous, Immune and Endocrine Function

▶ *Magnesium* – A deficiency in magnesium can result in chronic fatigue and some studies have shown good results with magnesium supplementation. Suggested use: at least 500 – 1000 mg daily in divided doses

▶ *Siberian ginseng (Eleutherococcus senticosus)* – In addition to supporting the adrenal glands and the stress response, Siberian ginseng has been shown to promote immune function by increasing natural killer cell activity and T-helper cells. *See AdrenaSense.*

Other important supplements to consider: a high-potency multivitamin, vitamin C and B vitamins, especially pantothenic acid which have all been shown to improve symptoms of CFS.

Lifestyle and Diet Modifications for Inflammation

▶ Avoid bad types of fats like saturated fats in red meats, dairy products, peanuts, pastries, muffins, trans fatty acids, hydrogenated oils and margarines. All of the fats in these products break down into compounds which increase pain and inflammation.
▶ Increase your intake of healthy fats like olive oil, fish oils and avocados as these fats help to reduce pain and inflammation. These foods can assist with arthritis, eczema, psoriasis, bursitis and all other inflammatory conditions.
▶ Avoid sugar as it increases insulin levels which serve only to increase inflammation and disease in the body. Consume low glycemic carbohydrates like whole grains, fruits, green vegetables, beans and oatmeal while avoiding sweets, candies, pop, pastries and baked goods as often as possible.

▸ Increase intake of spices like turmeric, rosemary and hops, as well as foods like pineapple and papaya. These all contain ingredients which are naturally anti-inflammatory.

▸ As mentioned previously in the CFS and FM sections, food allergies may be a hidden cause of chronic inflammation and immune system dysfunction. Food allergies are also linked to "leaky gut syndrome," a condition whereby damage to the gut lining allows large protein molecules to be absorbed into the bloodstream. The immune system then treats the molecules as foreign and starts making antibodies which results in inflammation and stress on the immune system. Known food allergens and foods than can be "pro-inflammatory" are red meat, saturated fats, dairy, gluten, egg, caffeine and alcohol, which all may worsen symptoms and should be eliminated.

▸ Members of the nightshade family such as tomatoes, potatoes, pepper and eggplant should also be eliminated or limited. They can increase inflammation in some individuals.

Nutritional Supplementation for Healthy Inflammatory Responses

▸ *Omega-3s:* EPA and DHA, the active constituents of fish oils, have anti-inflammatory effects. As a result, fish oil is used to help people with various inflammatory conditions. The EPA component holds especially potent anti-inflammatory properties useful for heart health and treating inflammatory conditions, while DHA is an important structural component of the brain, eyes and nervous system. Suggested use: a minimum of 1000 mg EPA and 500 mg DHA daily. For extreme inflammatory conditions, 3000-5000 mg of EPA can be taken daily.

▸ *Glucosamine sulfate, chondroitin sulfate and MSM:* Glucosamine is produced naturally in the body to help maintain and build healthy joint tissue that seems to fade with the aging process. Chondroitin sulfate is vital to the structure and function of cartilage as it provides it with shock absorption properties. MSM holds our basic connective tissues together, forming the elemental structure of proteins, and is required for a number of processes in our bodies. It also possesses a powerful anti-inflammatory effect.

▸ *Curcumin* (*Curcuma longa*) is a perennial herb - commonly known as turmeric, especially in its powdered form - that belongs to the ginger family. This spice is cancer protective, a potent antioxidant, supports liver function and is anti-inflammatory.

▶ *Celadrin®:* Celadrin works similar to essential fatty acids, EPA and DHA (from fish oils). It is a complex blend of esterified fatty acids which supports comfortable joint movement, flexibility and mobility. It also helps lubricate and cushion joints.
Suggested use: 3 softgels/day

▶ *AdrenaSense®:* Supporting the adrenal glands and the stress response is key to supporting the body's natural inflammatory responses.
Suggested use: 2 capsules midday with food

▶ *Devil's claw (Harpagophytum procumbens):* Extracts from the African plant devil's claw contain harpagosides – active compounds with potent anti-inflammatory, analgesic and anti-arthritic actions. Devil's claw has been shown to significantly reduce the pain and stiffness associated with arthritis.

▶ *Boswellia serrata:* Extracts of the plant *Boswellia serrata* have been noted for their anti-inflammatory properties and can be useful for the pain and stiffness associated with joint problems and rheumatoid arthritis.

▶ *Enzymes:* Plant-based digestive enzymes (bromelain, papain) and pancreatin enzymes (animal based) work as powerful anti-inflammatory agents, reducing pain, swelling and infection while improving joint flexibility.

CHAPTER 13

Twenty-Five Stress-Busting Recipes
by Julie Daniluk (RHN), Nutritionist, Author and
Television Host of *Healthy Gourmet*

 Julie Daniluk, RHN, hosts *Healthy Gourmet*, a reality cooking show that highlights the ongoing battle between taste and nutrition by using unique groups such as bikers, dragon boat racers and ballroom dancers to challenge their taste buds with nutritious foods. As a nutritional expert, Julie has appeared in over 300 TV and radio segments including City TV's *Perfect Fit*, *The Gill Deacon Show* on the CBC, CTV's *Balance* and *Three Takes* on Slice Network. Television viewers recognize her most from her "busted" segments on *The Right Fit* (W Network) where she examines the foods people need to purchase to stay healthy and grades healthy choices on restaurant menus, acting as a nutrition encyclopedia.

RECIPES TO START THE DAY

► Ultimate Quinoa Porridge

Rolled quinoa (pronounced keen-wa) is a wonderful alternative to oatmeal. Quinoa is a nutty gluten free grain that provides 8 grams of protein and 5 grams of fiber in 1 cooked cup and is a good natural source of iron. It also has good amounts of zinc, vitamin E and selenium to help control your weight and lower your risk of diabetes.

Ingredients:

1 cup (250 mL)	filtered water
1/3 cup (80 mL)	rolled quinoa
1 scoop	PGX® Satisfast™ Vegan Protein Shake
1/2 tsp (2.5 mL)	cinnamon
1/2 cup (125 mL)	berries
2 tbsp (30 mL)	hemp seeds

Optional: milk of choice (cow, goat, rice, almond)

Directions:

1 Boil the water in a small saucepan. Add the rolled quinoa and stir for 2 to 3 minutes.
2 Remove from heat and mix in the PGX® Satisfast™ Vegan Protein Shake, cinnamon, fruit and seeds until evenly distributed.
3 Top with choice of milk (cow, goat, rice, almond)

Makes 1 serving.

▶ Maca Berry Crisp

If your adrenals had a dream food, it would be maca. This cruciferous root not only has adaptogenic properties (which means it helps the body cope with stress by supporting adrenal health), but is also a brain tonic that helps decrease the release of ACTH (adrenocorticotropic hormone; *see page 9*). Maca is also a reproductive tonic, meaning it protects against stress-induced imbalances in sex hormones. This low glycemic index dessert is sweetened with sterol-rich mesquite powder and spiced with stress-busting cloves. Cloves help prevent stress-induced gastric ulcers, while also helping your body cope with the chemical fluctuations caused by stress.

Fruit-Base Ingredients:

6 cups (1.5 L)	organic fresh or frozen strawberries, halved
4 cups (1 L)	organic apples, sliced
3 cups (750 mL)	fresh organic peaches, sliced*
1/2 cup (125 mL)	organic goji berries
1 cup (250 mL)	unsweetened berry juice
2 tbsp (30 mL)	lemon juice
1/2 tsp (2.5 mL)	clove powder
1/2 tsp (2.5 mL)	nutmeg powder

Topping Ingredients:

1 cup (250 mL)	quinoa flakes
1/2 cup (125 mL)	brown rice flour
1/4 cup (60 mL)	hazelnuts, chopped
1/2 cup (125 mL)	maple syrup
1/3 cup (85 mL)	mesquite pod powder
2 tbsp (30 mL)	maca root powder
2 tsp (10 mL)	cinnamon powder
1/2 tsp (2.5 mL)	ginger powder
1/4 tsp (1 mL)	pink rock or gray sea salt
4 tbsp (60 mL)	cold coconut butter, cut into 8 pieces

Directions to make the fruit base:

1 Preheat the oven to 350°F.
2 In a medium bowl combine the strawberries, apples, peaches and goji berries.
3 Add the berry juice, lemon juice, cloves and nutmeg.
4 Toss thoroughly and transfer to a 9″ x 13″ baking dish.

Directions to make the topping:

1 In a large bowl, combine the quinoa flakes, brown rice flour, hazelnuts, maple syrup, mesquite powder, maca powder, cinnamon, ginger and sea salt. Place the coconut butter on top of the flour mixture. Using your hand, blend until the mixture looks like coarse meal.
2 Sprinkle the topping evenly and loosely over the fruit mixture, leaving fruit visible in a few spots for the juices to bubble up.
3 Transfer to the oven. Bake the crisp for 45 minutes or until the top is brown and the fruit juices are bubbling at the edges.

* Substitute with more organic apples if fresh peaches are not available.
Makes 8 servings.

▶ Eggs in the Bunny Hole

Just like Peter Rabbit, who loved to dig a hole in the vegetable patch, we are going to dig holes in this vegetable medley and poach our eggs over top to protect the lipid-rich yolk from oxidation. This is the perfect way to start your day. By eating a lot of protein in the morning, you are sure to have both stable moods and blood sugar to last you until lunchtime. You will find you have more focus to tackle life!

Three tablespoons of shiitake mushrooms pack more than 90% of your daily recommended intake of vitamin B5! Shiitake mushrooms are also a good source of other B vitamins, plus selenium and zinc, which keep your adrenal glands well nourished. Egg yolks are a superb source of lecithin, and gentle heating doesn't destroy this vital nutrient. Lecithin is a key element in all cell membranes and is especially important for nervous system function. Calm your nerves, and your adrenals will also be soothed.

Ingredients:

2 tsp (10 mL)	extra-virgin olive oil
1 clove	garlic, crushed and finely chopped
1/2 tsp (2.5 mL)	fresh basil, chopped
1/2 tsp (2.5 mL)	fresh oregano

1 cup (250 mL)	onion, chopped
2/3 cup (185 mL)	shiitake mushroom, chopped
1 cup (250 mL)	zucchini, chopped
1 cup (250 mL)	cherry tomatoes
4 large	eggs
to taste	pink rock or gray sea salt
2 tbsp (30 mL)	fresh parsley, chopped

Directions:

1   Heat a large cast iron skillet over medium heat. Add extra-virgin olive oil, garlic, basil and oregano.
2   Add the onion and shiitake mushroom. Cook, stirring occasionally, for 3 to 5 minutes or until tender.
3   Add the zucchini. Cook for about 2 more minutes. Add tomatoes and warm gently for 1 minute.
4   Dig 4 holes into the vegetable mixture, break eggs, and pour them into the holes. Cook until eggs reach desired consistency (about 3 more minutes). Keep in mind that a runny yolk is the healthiest, but egg whites are best when cooked thoroughly.
5   Transfer to dishes. Season to taste with sea salt and sprinkle chopped parsley over top.
6   Serve immediately.

Makes 2 servings.

▶ Carob Hazelnut Spread

Chocolate-hazelnut spread is one of the most decadent spreads you can eat on toast. However, if you're healing adrenal fatigue, you won't be able to toler-ate the caffeine-heavy chocolate or the refined carbohydrates in toast. Carob is an equally decadent alternative to chocolate-hazelnut spreads. It is a high-fiber bean that tastes uncannily like cacao. However, it contains no caffeine, so it won't exhaust your adrenal glands. Instead, it potentially will nourish your adrenals because carob is a good source of vitamins B2, B3 and B6, plus calcium, copper, manganese and potassium. Copper is used by the adrenals to help produce epinephrine and norepinephrine, while manganese is a critical component of the powerful antioxidant enzyme manganese superoxide dis-mutase, which is produced by the adrenal glands.

Ingredients:

2 whole	ripe avocados
4 whole	Medjool dates, soaked in 1/2 cup water
3 tbsp (45 mL)	carob bean powder
1 tsp (1 mL)	cinnamon powder
pinch	pink rock or gray sea salt

Recommended Flavor Variations:

1/4 to 1/2 tsp	ginger powder
1/4 tsp	clove powder
1/2 tsp	nutmeg powder
1 tsp	vanilla bean powder

Directions:

1 Combine all ingredients in a blender, including the 1/2 cup of water used to soak the dates.
2 Whip until smooth.
3 Serve immediately or store in a sealed glass jar or container for up to 3 days.

Makes 2 cups.

▶ Superfood Smoothies

Create your own solar-charged energy! Do you find that in the summer you just don't feel up to eating big meals? Consider making a cool smoothie instead and supply your body with readily available nutrition. Fresh vegetable juice and fruit smoothies don't just taste great – they help you enjoy more produce in a day than you would ever imagine!

It is best to eat fruits in a smoothie as opposed to juicing them, since you lose a lot of the important polyphenols that prevent cancer when you remove the skin. Also, the fiber in fruit is important for helping to stabilize blood sugar levels. Buy organic whenever you can, as delicate fruit is higher in pesticides, which are impossible to remove with washing.

Some fruits that mix well include:

Apple	Apricot
Blackberry	Cantaloupe
Cherry	Currants
Cranberry	Durian
Elderberry	Gooseberry

Grape	Grapefruit
Honeydew	Kiwi
Kumquat	Lemon
Lime	Lychee
Mandarin	Orange
Mango	Mangosteen
Orange	Papaya passion fruit
Peach	Pineapple
Pear	Pomegranate
Plum	Strawberry
Raspberry	Watermelon
Tangerine	

Why Organic is Always Better

A two-year review conducted in March 2008 by Charles Benbrook, Xin Zhao, Jaime Yanez, Neal Davies and Preston Andrews showed that organic produce is higher in nutrition.

The research team created a large database, which included the results of nearly one hundred well-designed studies that showed organically grown foods are 25% higher in nutrients than conventionally grown foods.

A big part of this increase is owing to the fact that plants use polyphenols (powerful antioxidants) to fight off pests and bacterial or fungal infections. If the plant is sprayed with pesticides and does not have to fight for itself, its need to produce the protective chemicals is reduced.

Check out the entire 53-page report at http://www.organic-center.org/science.nutri.php?action=view&report_id=126

If you are not using organically grown vegetables, always remove the peel. This helps to minimize your pesticide exposure. Unfortunately, much of the nutrients in vegetables are found within the peel.

VEGETABLE JUICES

Here is a list of vegetable choices that can be mixed and matched to create great tasting, healing beverages.

Alfalfa	Aloe vera
Artichoke	Arugula
Asparagus	Bamboo shoots

Basil

Beet greens

Bok choy

Brussels sprouts

Cabbage (red)

Cauliflower

Celery

Chinese cabbage (napa cabbage)

Collard greens

Cucumber

Endives

Garlic

Jicama

Kohlrabi

Lentil sprouts

Lettuce (radicchio)

Mung bean sprouts

Onions

Parsnip

Peppers (red)

Radishes

Scallions

Spinach

Sunflower sprouts

Tomatoes

Turnip greens

Wheat grass

Zucchini

Beet

Bitter melon (a type of gourd)

Broccoli

Cabbage (green)

Carrots

Celeriac

Chicory

Chives

Coriander

Dandelion leaves

Fennel

Ginger

Kale

Lamb's quarter

Lettuce (butter)

Lettuce (romaine)

Mustard greens

Parsley

Peppers (green)

Pumpkin

Radish sprouts

Spearmint (mint)

Stinging nettle

Swiss chard

Turnips

Watercress

Yams

Buying a Juicer

I suggest that you buy a juicer that is very easy to clean. When I first bought a juicer ten years ago, you needed a jet-engine mechanic to put it back together. I eventually sold it and am thrilled with my easy-to-clean, pressing-style juicer. A juice press in very important for three reasons:

1 Juice extracted with a press does not oxidize as quickly because a high-speed blade is not used to extract the juice. A juice press is basically a heavy-duty screw that presses the veggies or fruit against a metal screen.

2 Pressing preserves the greatest amount of enzymes in the juice. Because the press extracts slowly, it prevents the juice from heating up.

3 It is faster to use a press. Standard bucket-style juicers might seem faster because you can stick a whole apple or carrot in it without cutting it up first. The time you think you are saving is wasted in the end during clean up – the hundreds of holes in a large bucket screen are a complete pain to clean!

Two small notes about juice presses to ensure success:

1 Because presses do not have blades, it helps to alternate between soft and hard vegetables. Soft vegetables don't release their juice as fast as hard veggies. When you use a harder vegetable after a soft vegetable, you help to flush the juice from the soft one more easily into your glass.

2 When juicing small leaves like cilantro or parsley, wrap the leaves inside a bigger leaf vegetable such as kale, or roll the smaller leaves into a ball to maximize the yield.

Tips to keep in mind if you are just starting out:

1 Keep it simple. With simplicity comes consistency. If you make it a routine you can stick with, you are sure to see results.

2 Avoid the sugar daddy!

If you suffer from a sugar related health problem such as diabetes, hypoglycemia or heart disease it is important to stick to the green veggies and just add enough apple or carrot to help make it taste good. Let your health care professional know you want to start a juicing program so they can consult with you on how to adjust your medication.

For reduction of inflammation and correct hormone balance, you must keep your blood sugar in a narrow range. If you allow your blood sugar to get too high by eating lots of sugar and starches, you will promote inflammation. If you skip meals, you will risk producing more stress hormones and feelings of irritability. I have made the following recipes less sweet than those you may find in a juice bar, but this is important for adrenal healing. These juices are delicious and refreshing, yet nourishing – perfect on a hot summer day.

Rainbow Reason

We have all heard that it is smart to eat a rainbow of color, and there is a good reason why. By alternating the produce you juice, you get a wider spectrum of nutrition. This means that while one vegetable may be low in a certain vitamin or mineral, another vegetable may not. By eating (or in this case, drinking) a variety, you ensure complete nutrition. Variety also safeguards us from food sensitivities. If you eat the same food every day, you risk having your immune system flag that food as an allergen.

The following recipes do not have individual instructions. The process is very easy: just stick everything into the blender, make sure the lid is on tight, and blend until smooth. All recipes make 2 servings.

► Maca Piña Colada

The ingredients in this recipe will have your adrenals so pumped, you'll feel a natural energy "high" and you won't miss the alcohol. PGX® Satisfast™ Whey Protein is rich in high-quality whey protein. Maca has been traditionally used in Peru for hormone balance and fertility, and recent scientific studies show that this root can be a powerful tonic for the adrenal glands and reproductive organs. The coconut milk in this recipe will provide long-lasting fuel, and the freshly ground flax seeds will help stabilize your blood sugar levels because they are filled with fiber, essential fatty acids, protein and minerals. If that weren't enough, the easily digestible goat or sheep yogurt will support your digestive health by providing probiotics as well as short-chain fatty acids that support bowel flora. Who knew a virgin piña colada could be a nutritious meal and also provide adrenal support?

Ingredients:

1/2 cup (125 mL)	fresh pineapple, chopped
1/2 cup (125 mL)	pineapple juice
1/2 cup (125 mL)	filtered water
3/4 cup (185 mL)	goat or sheep yogurt
1/4 cup (60 mL)	coconut milk
2 scoops (34 g)	PGX® Satisfast™ Whey Protein Very Vanilla
1 tsp (5 mL)	flax seed, freshly ground
1 tsp (5 mL)	maca root powder

Makes 4 cups.

▸ Sprout to Life

Sprouts are live food – they contain every nutrient a body that is healing needs. Sprouting tends to make many nutrients more available for digestion and assimilation. Sunflower seed sprouts are rich in B vitamins and essential amino acids – precisely the nutrients your adrenal glands need to work at their optimum. The spirulina adds some detox support and blends nicely with PGX® Satisfast™ Whey Protein and sweet, fresh fruit. Cleansing your tissues is more important for stress reduction than many people realize. If your cells are struggling to function because they are full of toxins, then you will be less resilient to stress, be it psychological, physical or environmental.

Ingredients:

2 cups (500 mL)	filtered water
1 cup (250 mL)	pear juice
1 cup (250 mL)	fresh peaches, sliced
1/2 cup (125 mL)	sunflower seed sprouts
2 scoops (34 g)	PGX® Satisfast™ Whey Protein Very Vanilla
1 tbsp (15 mL)	spirulina powder

Makes 5 cups.

▸ Mulberry Magic

Your adrenal glands have a high metabolism – they are always working to regulate blood pressure, balance blood sugar, sustain energy and help orchestrate hormone activity throughout your body. This means they generate a vast number of free radicals and therefore need an equally massive arsenal of antioxidants to prevent cell damage. Fresh berries such as mulberries can come to the rescue. Mulberries are relentless free radical fighters, and they are also rich in minerals. In traditional Chinese medicine, mulberry fruits are esteemed as antistress rejuvenating tonics, similar to goji berries. Bananas are one of the best fruit sources of vitamin B6 – the nutrient that supports the synthesis of serotonin in the brain. Vitamin B6 is involved in the production of adrenal hormones and helps balance the activity of steroid hormones.

Ingredients:

2 cups (500 mL)	filtered water
1 cup (250 mL)	fresh mulberries, or 1/3 cup (85 mL) dried mulberries soaked in 2/3 cup (175 mL) filtered water

1/4 cup (60 mL)	coconut milk
1 whole	frozen banana
1 tbsp (15 mL)	tiger nut powder
1 tsp (5 mL)	inulin fiber
1/4 tsp (1 mL)	cinnamon powder

Makes 4 cups.

▸ Hippy Hippy Shake

Imagine a delicious, sweet food that is rich in omega-6 essential fatty acids and artery lubricating omega-9s; insulin supporting chromium; blood-building iron; an alkalizing and nerve nourishing calcium-magnesium combination with an almost perfect 2:1 ratio; immune- and adrenal-supporting zinc; antioxidant selenium; cleansing fiber; and the full spectrum of your daily recommended intake of each essential amino acid. If it were possible, your adrenals would be drooling right now! Your pancreas and liver would also be rejoicing because this low glycemic treat is also safe for diabetics. You're probably wondering if such a wonder food actually exists. The good news is that it does! Tiger nuts (*Cyperus esculentus*), which are actually sedge tubers, have been used in traditional medicine as a digestive tonic and recent studies suggest they help prevent colon cancer. They give this shake a uniquely delicious taste and satisfying richness. The cinnamon bite not only stimulates your digestive juices, but also regulates your blood sugar because of the way it helps insulin do its job. This shake is a wonderful celebration of flavors. It's a perfect energy boost first thing in the morning and a fabulous pick-me-up snack between meals.

Ingredients:

1 large	apple, chopped
3 whole	Medjool dates, pitted
1/3 cup (85 mL)	hemp seeds
1/4 cup (60 mL)	almonds
1/2 tsp (2.5 mL)	cinnamon powder
1/2 tsp (1 mL)	ginger powder

Recommended Ingredients:

| 2 tbsp (30 mL) | tiger nut powder |
| 1 tsp (5 mL) | mesquite pod powder |

Makes 4 cups.

▶ **Lemonade High**

You may think you can't make it through the day without your morning (and perhaps afternoon!) cup of coffee. The truth is, your adrenals loathe this caffeine-drenched stimulant. Caffeine mercilessly kicks your adrenals into full action – whether or not they're ready for the front lines! Chances are, if you feel lifeless without caffeine, then your adrenals are equally drained of vitality. It may seem that you have no alternative, but this delicious lemonade is actually an energizing adrenal elixir!

Ginseng roots are prized for their adrenal tonic properties and, as such, are famous as life-extending herbs. The most commonly used species are red Korean (*Panax ginseng*) and American (*Panax quinquefolius*) ginseng. Siberian ginseng (*Eleutherococcus senticosus*, commonly known as eleuthero) is no longer considered a true ginseng even though its medicinal properties are very similar to the Panax species. Powdered codonopsis root (*Codonopsis pilosula*), also known as dang shen or poor man's ginseng, can also be substituted in this recipe. As its name suggests, it is much less expensive than the true ginsengs, but fortunately it is equally effective in toning the adrenals. The true ginsengs can be quite stimulating, so introduce them into your diet gradually. You can start by replacing your morning coffee or black tea with this super-charged, detoxifying, adrenal-invigorating lemonade. Alternatively, you can choose eleuthero or codonopsis, as they are gentler and less stimulating.

Amla (*Phyllanthus emblica*) is Indian gooseberry. It is one of the fundamental whole body tonics in Ayurvedic medicine, prized for its ability to help rejuvenate cells and restore health. This tart fruit is brimming with vitamin C, bioflavonoids and antioxidants, which are healing to your glands.

Ingredients:

4 cups (1 L)	filtered water
1	organic lemon
1 tsp (5 g)	glutamine powder
1/2 tsp (2.5 mL)	amla berry powder or rose hip powder
1/2 tsp (2.5 mL)	ginseng root powder or liquid tincture
10 drops (1 mL)	stevia liquid extract or 1 tbsp (15 mL) raw honey

Directions:

1 Place filtered water in a blender.
2 Peel the lemon, leaving some of the healthy white rind, as it is full of antioxidant bioflavonoids. Cut into chunks and remove seeds.
3 Add the glutamine powder, amla or rose hip powder, ginseng root and stevia extract or honey.

4 Blend on high until smooth. Enjoy!

Makes 4 cups.

▶ Licorice Lemonade

Licorice is an incredible herb that tones and strengthens the adrenals glands. It contains well over 150 compounds, including an extremely active compound known as glycyrrhizin (or glycyrrhizic acid). While glycyrrhizin is very healing to the adrenal glands, it does cause a rise in blood pressure. People who suffer from hypertension should therefore avoid licorice or consume deglycyrrhizinated forms that don't affect blood pressure.

Glutamine is an amino acid that becomes conditionally essential during periods of stress or infection. Your body – especially the cells of your digestive tract, adrenal glands and immune system – thrives when this amino acid is abundant. What better way to show your adrenals you love them than with this lively lemonade?

Ingredients:

4 cups (1 L)	filtered water
1	organic lemon
1 tsp (5 g)	glutamine powder
1/2 tsp (2.5 mL)	licorice solid extract
10 drops (1 mL)	stevia liquid extract or 1 tbsp (15 mL) raw honey

Directions:

1 Place filtered water in a blender.

2 Peel the lemon, leaving some of the healthy white rind, as it is full of antioxidant bioflavonoids. Cut into chunks and remove seeds.

3 Add the glutamine powder, licorice and stevia or honey.

4 Blend on high until smooth. Enjoy!

CAUTION: Avoid concentrated licorice extract if you suffer from hypertension as it can elevate blood pressure. Consult your health care practitioner before you use licorice extract/syrup or powder.

Makes 4 cups.

EASY LUNCHES

▶ Healthy Homemade Dijon-Mayo

You'll be amazed at the bright flavor of homemade mayonnaise. It's really very simple and fast to make with a blender or processor. It's even nutritious – who would have thought? Eggs contain stress-busting choline, a chemical precursor or "building block" needed to produce the neurotransmitter acetylcholine. Research suggests that memory, intelligence and mood are mediated at least in part by acetylcholine metabolism in the brain.

Ingredients:

2	egg yolks
3/4 tsp (4 mL)	gray sea salt
1/2 tsp (2.5 mL)	mustard powder
1/4 tsp (1 mL)	honey
4 to 5 tsp (20 to 25 mL)	lemon juice
1 cup (250 mL)	extra-virgin olive oil, divided
4 tsp	filtered water, heated

Directions:

1   Beat egg yolks with sea salt, mustard, honey and 1 tsp (5 mL) of lemon juice in a small bowl until very thick and pale yellow. (Note: If using electric mixer, beat at medium speed.)
2   Add about 1/4 cup (60 mL) extra-virgin olive oil, little by little, beating vigorously all the while. Beat in 1 tsp (5 mL) each lemon juice and hot water.
3   Add another 1/4 cup (60 mL) extra-virgin olive oil, a few drops at a time, while beating vigorously. Beat in another tsp (5 mL) each of lemon juice and hot water.
4   Add remaining 1/2 cup (125 mL) extra-virgin olive oil in a very fine steady stream, beating constantly. Then mix in remaining lemon juice and hot water. If you prefer your mayonnaise thick and creamy, add a total of 4 tsp of lemon juice; if you prefer it light and tangy, add a total of 5 tsp.
5   Cover and refrigerate until needed. Consume within 1 week.

Makes 1-1/2 cups.

▶ **Asparagus and Salmon Rolls**

Asparagus is brimming with B vitamins that sustain your nerves during times of stress. One cup of raw asparagus also boasts 3 grams of protein, vitamin C, fiber and tissue repairing manganese and iron!

Chronic stress is a major source of inflammation, and omega-3 essential fatty acids act as powerful anti-inflammatory nutrients. Salmon is one of the richest sources of omega-3s, and the fish omegas docosahexaenoic acid (DHA) and eicosapentaenoic acid (EPA) are especially important for helping to minimize the amount of cortisol and epinephrine released during stress. Capers are among the highest sources of quercetin, an antioxidant nutrient that curbs your body from launching a disproportionately large fight-or-flight response when faced with stress.

Ingredients:

1 to 2 bunches	thin asparagus
1 tbsp	organic lemon juice
2 tbsp (50 mL)	Healthy Homemade Dijon-Mayo (see recipe page 118)
1 tsp (5 mL)	mustard powder
1 tbsp (15 mL)	pickled capers, chopped
200 g	nitrate-free smoked salmon
1 bunch	fresh chives
12	dry rice-paper rounds or whole collard leaves, de-stemmed and soaked in warm filtered water for 30 minutes

Directions:

Assembly:

1 Partially fill a large frying pan with 1" filtered water and bring to a boil over high heat.

2 Add asparagus and steam until tender-crisp, about 2 minutes. Drain and rinse under cold water to stop cooking.

3 Grate lemon zest and put aside.

4 In a small bowl, squeeze 1 tbsp (15 mL) lemon juice and then stir in mayonnaise and mustard powder. Add capers.

5 Fill a pie plate with lukewarm water and place beside a cutting board.

6 Line up smoked salmon, mayo mixture, lemon zest, asparagus and chives near cutting board.

7 Dip 1 rice-paper round at a time into water and let sit until very pliable, about 30 seconds, and then gently lay on a towel to dry. If using collard leaves, remove from water and pat dry with a clean cloth.

8   Place rice paper or soaked collard leaf on a cutting board.

9   Tear a slice of smoked salmon in half and place along the bottom third of the rice paper round or collard leaf.

10   Spread 1 tsp (5 mL) of mayo mixture over salmon.

11   Lay 4 asparagus spears over salmon.

12   Top with 4 or 5 chives.

Rolling:

1   Lift rice paper or collard leaf edge closest to you up and over the filling, and then roll tightly toward the center.

2   When you reach the center, fold in sides. Continue rolling to form a log.

3   To seal, dip a finger in water and rub over seam.

4   Set the roll seam-side down on a platter.

5   Repeat with remaining ingredients.

6   Serve immediately or cover and refrigerate up to 4 hours.

7   Before serving, slice rolls in half diagonally and serve.

Note: If rice-paper rounds curl before being soaked, don't worry. They will flatten when they are placed in water. As the soaking water cools, replace with lukewarm water.

Makes 12 servings.

▸ Miami Salad

If you live in a climate with a cold winter, it's easy to forget fresh fruits, vegetables and salads because you crave cooked comfort foods instead. This easy-to-make, refreshing salad provides plenty of fiber and carotenoids thanks to the raw ingredients it contains. Avocados are very high in vitamin B5 (also known as pantothenic acid), which is essential for adrenal health. This vitamin makes the adrenals more sensitive to ACTH (adrenocorticotropic hormone; *see page 17*) and helps to prevent the adrenals from releasing excess amounts of cortisol under stress. It is also vital to sustaining adrenal tissue health and for synthesizing adrenal hormones.

Apple cider vinegar helps to regulate your blood-sugar levels, and so protects your adrenals from having to release epinephrine when blood glucose drops too low. Grapefruit packs vitamin C, while spinach boosts your vitamin A levels – two vitamins that nourish your adrenals.

Salad Ingredients:

2 medium	pink grapefruit, pared
4 cups (1 L)	baby spinach
1 medium	avocado, peeled and sliced
2 medium (280 g)	cooked chicken breasts, seasoned and sliced

or vegan option:

1-1/2 cups (325 mL)	aduki beans, cooked or one 14-oz (400 mL) can, drained and rinsed

Dressing Ingredients:

2 tbsp (30 mL)	extra-virgin olive oil
1 tbsp (15 mL)	flax seed oil
2 tsp (10 mL)	unpasteurized apple cider vinegar
2 tsp (10 mL)	fresh basil, chopped
1/4 tsp (1 mL)	pink rock or gray sea salt

Directions:

1 Using a small sharp knife, section grapefruit over a small bowl to catch juices.
2 Place spinach in a large bowl.
3 Alternately arrange grapefruit and avocado slices with sliced chicken or aduki beans over top.
4 To prepare dressing, add all ingredients to the small bowl containing grapefruit juice. Whisk and then pour dressing evenly over the salad.
5 Serve immediately.

Makes 2 servings.

▶ French-Mint White-Bean Dip

This dip is so rich in flavor that you can easily slip in a dose of adrenal maca-medicine without altering the taste. Beans are a delicious source of folic acid, which may improve depression, possibly because it is essential for the production of red blood cells. An oxygen-deprived brain can lead to emotional and psychological imbalances, which signal a stress response in the whole body. Rosemary and mint are also used as antidepressants because they stimulate blood circulation, and therefore, oxygen delivery to the brain. You can quickly whip up this dip to enjoy a brain- and adrenal-tonic meal.

Ingredients:

2 cups (500 mL)	white kidney or navy beans, cooked or one 19-oz (560 mL) can, drained and rinsed
1/4 cup (60 mL)	extra-virgin olive oil
3 tbsp (30 mL)	freshly squeezed lemon juice
2 tbsp (30 mL)	fresh mint
1 tbsp (15 mL)	maca powder
1 tsp (5 mL)	fresh rosemary
1/4 tsp (1 mL)	pink rock or gray sea salt
1 tbsp (15 mL)	fresh parsley, finely chopped

Recommended Ingredient:

1/2 tsp (2.5 mL)	spirulina powder

Directions:

1 In a food processor or blender, combine all ingredients except the parsley. Purée until smooth.
2 Place in a serving dish and garnish with parsley.
3 Serve immediately or cover and refrigerate for up to 3 days. Before serving, bring to room temperature and check seasoning.

Makes 2-1/2 cups.

▶ Almond-Butter Greens

Rich and creamy almond butter is a delectable way to nourish your adrenals. It makes steamed greens come alive. It packs an incredible amount of magnesium, which helps soothe your adrenals and nerves – you'll get an awesome 95% of your daily recommended intake in 1/2 cup of almond butter! The high potassium content of this nut also helps your adrenals because vast amounts of this essential mineral are required for proper adrenal functioning (particularly for synthesizing and releasing adrenal hormones).

The adrenals also help regulate the balance of sodium and potassium in the blood. They secrete a hormone called aldosterone that signals the kidneys to release potassium in the urine while reabsorbing sodium. High sodium diets, which are often a result of eating mostly table salt that is devoid of potassium, can lead to electrolyte imbalances, as well as hyperstimulation of the adrenal glands. Sea salt and potassium-rich foods such as almonds can help restore this essential electrolyte.

Greens Ingredients:

8 cups	chard, spinach, kale, or beet greens

Dressing Ingredients:

1/2 cup (125 mL)	almond butter
4 tbsp (60 mL)	filtered water
2 tbsp (30 mL)	umeboshi vinegar
1 tbsp (15 mL)	raw honey with propolis and/or royal jelly
1 tsp (5 mL)	nutritional yeast

Directions:

1 Place washed greens in a stainless steel steaming basket over a pot containing a small amount of boiling filtered water. Cover with a lid. Steam 2 minutes for spinach, 3 minutes for chard and beet greens, and 5 minutes for kale.
2 Transfer steamed greens to a large bowl and let cool slightly.
3 Combine all the dressing ingredients in a cup and mix well with a fork.
4 Pour sauce over the greens and enjoy while still warm. Leftovers can be stored in a sealed glass jar or container in the fridge for up to a week.

Makes 3 to 4 servings plus an additional 1/2 cup dressing.

▶ Fennel-Ginger Salad

The avocado, hazelnuts, flax oil and hemp seeds in this recipe provide all the vitamin E your adrenals could want in one meal. Your adrenals store the highest concentration of vitamin E of all your organs, which shows the importance of this antioxidant for maintaining stress resilience.

This delicious sauce delivers the medicinal properties of umeboshi plums, which have been used as digestive and adrenal tonics in Asian traditional medicine for centuries. Umeboshi plums, also known as Japanese apricots, help your body deal with stress by restoring levels of adrenal epinephrine and norepinephrine following a stressful experience. Be careful not to use too much of this paste, as it's quite high in sea salt. I've added nutritional yeast to this recipe because it gives every dish a rich, buttery taste that is irresistible – even kids love it! More importantly, all the B vitamins, chromium, germanium, potassium, selenium and zinc found in nutritional yeast make it an adrenal superfood.

Salad Ingredients:

4 cups (1000 mL)	sliced fennel or celery
1/2 cup (125 mL)	green onion, thinly sliced
1/2 cup (125 mL)	hazelnuts, coarsely chopped
1 large	tangerine, peeled and sectioned
1 large	pear, cubed
1 large	apple, cubed
1 large	ripe avocado

Dressing Ingredients:

1/4 cup (60 mL)	pickled ginger, chopped
2 tbsp (30 mL)	coconut milk or Healthy Homemade Dijon-Mayo (*see recipe on page 118*)
2 tbsp (30 mL)	flax or hemp seed oil
1 tsp (5 mL)	umeboshi plum paste or 1/2 tsp (2.5 mL) sea salt, or to taste

Directions:

1 Combine salad ingredients in a large bowl.

2 In a cup, whisk together dressing ingredients. Pour over salad.

3 Toss gently and serve immediately.

Makes 8 servings.

▶ Stress Busting Dip

Lima beans are a good source of the trace essential mineral molybdenum. Molybdenum plays a huge role in supporting liver detoxification of adrenal hormones. It's important that your liver clears adrenal hormones from your bloodstream once they have done their job, otherwise they will continue to stimulate your body even after the stressful stimulus is gone. The essential-fatty-acid-rich flaxseed oil and hemp seeds will strengthen your brain/adrenal gland connection and improve your ability to adapt to stress. Flax seeds are high in omega-3s, whereas hemp seeds are high in omega-6s and extra-virgin olive oil supplies omega-9s. With this nutritious dip, your adrenals get the best of all healing fats in a balanced anti-inflammatory ratio.

Ingredients:

2-1/4 cups (560 mL)	lima beans, cooked or one 19-oz (560 mL) can, drained and rinsed

1/2 cup (125 mL)	lemon juice
1/2 cup (125 mL)	hemp seeds
1/2 cup (125 mL)	sunflower seeds
1/2 cup (125 mL)	flaxseed oil
1/4 cup (60 mL)	extra-virgin olive oil
1/4 cup (60 mL)	filtered water
1 tsp (5 mL)	dry basil
1/2 tsp (2.5 mL)	pink rock or gray sea salt

Recommended Ingredient:

1/2 tsp	nutritional yeast

Directions:
1 Mix all ingredients in a food processor with the S-blade. Blend for 5 to 7 minutes or until extra-creamy.
2 Serve immediately or store in a sealed glass jar or container for no more than 4 days.

Makes 3 cups.

▸ Sunny Sunflower Pâté

This pâté is another delicious way to boost your adrenals' levels of vitamin E. Your adrenals store ten times more vitamin E than any other organ. Since this fat-soluble vitamin is also essential for cardiovascular and nervous system health, you should make sure to eat at least your daily recommended intake of 15 mg (22 IU) from whole foods each day. The sunflower seeds, hemp seeds and extra-virgin olive oil in this recipe will satisfy your adrenals' hunger for this antioxidant vitamin.

Ingredients:

1 cup (250 mL)	raw sunflower seeds, soaked
1 cup (250 mL)	raw hemp seeds, hulled
1/2 cup (125 mL)	dill weed, chopped
2 tbsp (30 mL)	filtered water
2 tbsp (30 mL)	cold-pressed raw flax seed oil
2 tbsp (30 mL)	red onion or scallions, minced
2 tbsp (30 mL)	lemon juice
2 cloves	garlic
1/2 tsp (2.5 mL)	pink rock or gray sea salt

| 1/2 tsp (2.5 mL) | turmeric powder |
| 1/2 tsp (2.5 mL) | cumin powder |

Directions:

1   Place all ingredients in the food processor, using the S-blade to blend until paste-like.
2   Serve immediately or store in a sealed glass jar or container for up to a week.

Makes 4 servings.

LIGHT DINNERS

▶ Star Pho

Pho is a delicious Vietnamese soup typically made with rice noodles, meat and loads of leafy greens and herbs. The soup is richly flavored with anti-inflammatory spices and vegetables that will nourish almost every organ in your body. For example, one cup of amaranth leaves contains a whopping 400% of the daily recommended intake of vitamin K. Vitamin K helps the body recover from stress because it helps to repair tissue damage caused by long-term exposure to adrenal hormones. Vitamin K strengthens bones, supports vascular health, prevents oxidative damage, especially in nerve tissue, and helps heal skin hyperpigmentation. This meal is easy to digest yet satisfying enough to prevent you from overeating. If you make the stock ahead, it takes only minutes to prepare.

Spice Blend Ingredients:

3 whole	cloves
2 whole	star anise buds
1 strip (3 inches/8 cm long)	lime rind
1/2 tsp (3 mL)	coriander seeds

Soup Ingredients:

4 cups (1 L)	MSG-free beef or veggie stock
2 cups (500 mL)	filtered water
1 large	onion, chopped
2 cloves	garlic, smashed
3 thick slices	ginger root
8 oz (250 g)	skinless and boneless chicken thighs

or vegan option:

8 oz (250 g)	tempeh
4 cups (1 L)	amaranth leaf or baby bok choy, finely chopped
1 cup (250 mL)	mung bean sprouts
2 tbsp (30 mL)	lime juice
4 oz (120 g)	thin brown-rice noodles

Garnish Ingredients:

1/3 cup (85 mL)	fresh cilantro, chopped
2 tbsp (30 mL)	fresh mint, chopped
2 large	green onions, chopped

Directions:

1 In the center of a 6-inch (15 cm) double-thick square of cheesecloth, place cloves, star anise, lime rind and coriander seeds. Pull up corners and tie into a bundle with string. If you don't have cheesecloth, try using a paper filter.

2 In a large soup pot, add stock, water, onion, garlic, ginger root and spice bundle. Bring to a boil, then reduce heat and simmer for 10 minutes.

3 Thinly slice chicken or tempeh. Add to the boiling stock. If using chicken, skim off any foam with a spoon. Reduce heat and simmer for 15 minutes.

4 Meanwhile, in pot of boiling salted water, cook rice noodles until tender but firm, about 3 minutes; drain.

5 Divide greens (amaranth or baby bok choy) and noodles among 4 soup bowls. Top with bean sprouts.

6 Pour chicken or tempeh soup over greens, noodles and bean sprouts.

7 Garnish with mint, cilantro and green onions. Serve immediately.

Makes 4 servings.

▸ Spaghetti Squash and Turkey "Pasta"

Turkey is a great source of the amino acid tryptophan, which is a precursor to the relaxing neurotransmitter serotonin. It is also high in the amino acid tyrosine, which is a precursor to other neurotransmitters and hormones, including epinephrine, norepinephrine and dopamine. Supplying your adrenal glands with the nutrients they need to function will help prevent adrenal exhaustion.

Tomatoes are bursting with vitamin C, the antioxidant that not only protects your adrenals from free radical damage but also plays a role in the production of adrenal hormones and in the adrenals' stress response. Healing vitamin A from the pumpkin and spaghetti squash will boost cell-energy production and support your tissues during and after stressful periods. Cilantro is a delicious topper to this nutrient-dense dish and is a powerful, detoxifying, medicinal herb that helps to cleanse the body of adrenal-poisoning heavy metals.

Spaghetti Squash Ingredients:

1 large	spaghetti squash
2 tbsp (5 mL)	extra-virgin olive oil
to taste	pink rock or gray sea salt
1/2 lb (225 g)	green beans, blanched
2 cups (500 mL)	cherry tomatoes
2 small or 1 medium	zucchini, julienned
1 cup (250 mL)	fresh basil
2 cups (500 mL)	cilantro, finely chopped

Directions:

1 Preheat oven to 375 °F.
2 Cut squash in half horizontally and scoop out the seeds. Drizzle with 1 tbsp olive oil and season with sea salt.
3 Place squash on a baking sheet and roast cut-side down for approximately 1 hour.
4 Separate stems and leaves from basil. Set stems aside for use in turkey sauce and place leaves in a small bowl to use as garnish for final dish.
5 When squash is cooked, use a fork to pull strands away from the sides. Place "spaghetti" strands in a large serving bowl.
6 Fill a pot with one inch filtered water and bring to a gentle boil. Turn off heat, add green beans, and toss gently for 1 minute. Drain and rinse under cool water.
7 Add blanched green beans, cherry tomatoes and zucchini to the squash. Drizzle with 1 tbsp of extra-virgin olive oil and season with sea salt.
8 Top with turkey sauce, stir in cilantro and garnish with coarsely chopped basil leaves.

Turkey Sauce Ingredients:

1 large	onion, diced
2 cloves	garlic, crushed
1 tbsp (15 mL)	extra-virgin olive oil
to taste	pink rock and gray sea salt
1 lb (454 g)	ground turkey
1 bottle	whole peeled tomatoes
1 cup (250 mL)	fresh basil stems (separated from leaves; used as dish garnish)
1/2 cup (125 mL)	pumpkin puree

Directions:

1 In a saucepan, gently warm onions and garlic with extra-virgin olive oil. Sprinkle with sea salt to taste.

2 Add ground turkey and brown.

3 Crush tomatoes using your hands and add to pan with browned turkey.

4 Simmer for 30 minutes on low heat with basil stems (save basil leaves for later).

5 Add pumpkin puree and stir until blended.

Makes 6 servings.

▶ Oriental Turkey Salad

This salad is packed with protein – almonds, sesame seeds and turkey or black beans. Protein helps stabilize your blood sugar, which helps prevent adrenal strain. The amino acid tyrosine is especially important for your adrenals because it is a major building block for synthesizing epinephrine and norepinephrine. Most varieties of seaweed provide all the essential minerals your body needs for supporting enzyme activity, repairing tissues, and keeping hormones balanced. For example, sea vegetables are especially rich in iodine, which is key for supporting thyroid function. Without a balanced thyroid, your adrenals can't function at their best, and without balanced adrenals, your thyroid can't work at its optimum.

Salad Ingredients:

1/2 cup (125 mL)	whole raw almonds
1/2 pound (270g)	cooked boneless turkey breast, sliced into half inch strips

or vegan option:

1-3/4 cups (400 mL)	black beans, cooked or one 14-oz (400 mL) can, drained and rinsed
5 cups (1-1/4 L)	Chinese cabbage, thinly sliced
2 cups (500 mL)	Chinese long bean, chopped and steamed (or green beans)
1/2 cup (125 mL)	carrot, shredded
1/2 cup (125 mL)	green onion, chopped
1/4 cup (60 mL)	fresh cilantro, finely chopped
1/2 cup (125 mL)	seaweed flakes or wakame strips soaked in lemon and warm filtered water
2 tbsp (30 mL)	black or white raw sesame seeds

Dressing Ingredients:

2 tbsp (30 mL)	extra-virgin olive oil
2 tbsp (30 mL)	tamari soy sauce
1/4 cup (60 mL)	rice vinegar or unpasteurized apple cider vinegar
3 tbsp (45 mL)	raw honey, softened
1 tsp (1 mL)	red pepper flakes
1/2 tsp (2.5 mL)	pink rock or gray sea salt

Directions:

1 On a cutting board and using a sharp knife, carefully slice almonds. Toss into a large bowl.

2 Slice turkey strips and add the remaining salad ingredients, except for the sesame seeds.

3 In a small cup, whisk together extra-virgin olive oil, tamari sauce, vinegar, honey, red pepper flakes and sea salt.

4 Pour dressing over salad and toss gently. Sprinkle with sesame seeds.

Makes 2 servings.

▸ Black-Bean Bowl with Resto Pesto

As a young child, you may have been given cookies and milk to help you get to sleep. Milk relaxes you and helps you sleep because it is rich in melatonin, the neurotransmitter that signals "bedtime" to your brain. Numerous plants also contain melatonin and are excellent foods to eat when stress starts to cause anxiety or insomnia. Brown rice and garlic are especially rich in melatonin and will soothe your mind as does milk. The magnesium in the black beans, amaranth leaves and pesto will gently relax your nerves and muscles to ease any tension. Likewise, flax seed oil will quell inflammation in your nervous system and adrenals, calming you.

Ingredients:

1-1/2 cups (325 mL)	black beans, cooked or one 14-oz (400 mL) can, drained and rinsed
1/4 cup (125 mL)	Resto Pesto (see recipe on page 131 or use store-bought dairy-free pesto)
1/4 tsp (1 mL)	pink rock or gray sea salt
2 cups (500 mL)	brown rice, wild rice, quinoa or millet, cooked
4 small bunches	amaranth leaves, chopped or 4 cups (1 L) organic baby spinach, chopped

Recommended Ingredient:

2 tbsp (30 mL)	flax seed or extra-virgin olive oil (not needed if pesto is oily)

Directions:

1 In a bowl, gently mix the black beans with pesto and sea salt until well mixed.

2 In two serving bowls or portable containers, equally portion your grain of choice (brown rice, wild rice, quinoa or millet). Follow with chopped amaranth leaves (or baby spinach) and pesto beans. Drizzle with oil and season with additional salt and pepper if you think it's needed.

Makes 2 servings.

▶ Resto Pesto

Here's a pesto that will please your taste buds while it helps cleanse heavy metals from your bloodstream! Cilantro, chlorella and garlic are all well known for their ability to clear heavy metals from tissues. Flax oil and walnuts will supply essential fatty acids plus vitamin E to help minimize inflammation while you're cleansing, and the vitamin C plus bioflavonoids from the lemon juice will help protect your tissues. Heavy metals poison your adrenal glands and nervous system – especially your brain – so it's important to support daily removal of these toxins to prevent their accumulation in your tissues. Make sure you use the freshest ingredients available to make this antioxidant-rich pesto work wonders for you!

2 cups (500 mL)	fresh basil
2 cups (500 mL)	fresh cilantro
2 cups (500 mL)	raw kale
1 cup (250 mL)	whole walnuts
1 cup (250 mL)	flax seed oil
2 tbsp (30 mL)	umeboshi plum paste
2 tbsp (30 mL)	lemon juice, freshly squeezed
3 cloves	garlic
1/2 tsp (2.5 mL)	chlorella powder
1/4 tsp (1 mL)	pink rock or gray sea salt

Directions:

1 Put all ingredients in a blender or food processor. Blend on high until desired paste consistency is reached.

2   Store in an air-tight glass jar in your fridge for up to 2 weeks or in your freezer for up to 6 months.

Makes 3 cups.

▶ Jicama & Carrot Salad in Radicchio Cups

Jicama is my favorite veggie. It tastes like a pear and water chestnut in one. This salad can be enjoyed raw in the summer; however, blanching the ingredients makes the dish easier to digest for most people who are sensitive to raw foods. Jicama provides more than 50% of the daily recommended intake of vitamin C per serving, which replenishes your adrenal glands' supply of this essential antioxidant.

Ingredients:

7 medium (450 g)	carrots, peeled and cut into 2-inch long (5 cm) matchsticks
1 extra large (900 g)	jicama root, peeled and cut into 2-inch long (5 cm) matchsticks*
to taste	pink rock or gray sea salt
16 large	radicchio leaves (from about 2 heads), separated
16 to 32	fresh parsley sprigs

Dressing Ingredients:

1 large	green onion, minced
1 clove	garlic, minced
2/3 cup (185 mL)	hemp seeds
1 tsp (5 mL)	dijon mustard
3 tbsp (45 mL)	unpasteurized apple cider vinegar
2 tbsp (30 mL)	Healthy Homemade Dijon-Mayo (*see recipe on page 118*)
2 tbsp (30 mL)	fresh parsley, chopped
1/4 cup (60 mL)	extra-virgin olive oil

* Substitute with celery root if jicama is unavailable.

Directions:

1   Bring a large pot of salted water to a rolling boil.
2   Add carrot sticks and blanch for 1 minute or until tender-crisp. Drain and cool. Place into a small bowl. If you suffer from digestive problems, consider blanching the carrots and jicama until tender to ease digestion.
3   In a small cup, whisk together green onion, garlic, hemp seeds, mustard, vinegar, Healthy Mayo and parsley.

4 Add extra-virgin olive oil in a steady stream, whisking until combined.

5 Pour dressing over carrots and jicama. Toss and season with sea salt to taste.

6 To arrange, place a radicchio leaf in your hand and stuff the center with salad filling. Repeat with the remaining radicchio leaves, dividing the filling equally.

7 Garnish each with 1 to 2 parsley sprigs.

Makes 8 servings.

A FINAL TREAT

▶ Royal Halva

Your adrenals need magnesium and calcium to help regulate the release of epinephrine and norepinephrine, while your nerves need magnesium to relax and calcium to stimulate activity. Sesame seeds are an excellent source of both minerals. Royal jelly has long been regarded as an adrenal superfood because it is a top source of B vitamins and is high in protein. It also stimulates nerve-cell growth, which is important for recovering from stress.

Ingredients:

1 cup (250 mL)	black or white raw sesame seeds
1/4 cup (60 mL)	tahini (sesame seed butter)
1/4 cup (60 mL)	raw honey with added bee pollen or royal jelly
1 tbsp (15 mL)	chia or flax seeds, freshly ground
1/4 tsp (1 mL)	pink rock or gray sea salt

Recommended Adrenal Superfood Ingredient:

1 tsp (5 mL)	royal jelly

Directions:

1 Combine all ingredients in a food processor. Purée until smooth. If using, add extra royal jelly last to prevent oxidation. Pulse mixture briefly.

2 Line a container with a tight-fitting lid with parchment paper.

3 Press mixture into the container with the back of a spoon until tightly packed.

4 Cut into squares and place in fridge or freezer to set.

5 Consume directly from the container to prevent crumbling and immediately return to fridge or freezer to preserve the nutrients.

Makes 12 squares.

NOTES: